THE DIRECTORY OF
COMPLEMENTARY
THERAPIES

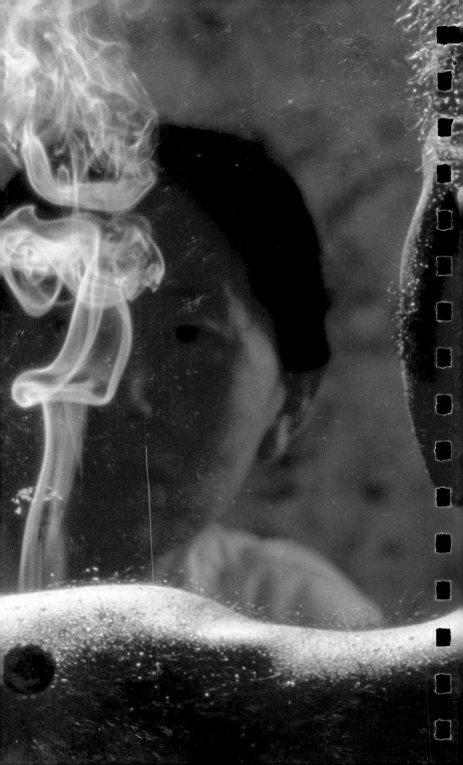

THE DIRECTORY OF
COMPLEMENTARY
THERAPIES

CONSULTANT EDITOR

C. NORMAN SHEALY, MD, PHD

CHARTWELL
BOOKS, INC.

First published in the United States in 2002 by
CHARTWELL BOOKS, INC.
A Division of Book Sales, Inc.
114 Northfield Avenue
Edison, New Jersey 08837

ISBN: 0–7858–1458–2

This book was conceived, designed, and produced by
THE IVY PRESS LIMITED
The Old Candlemakers, West Street,
Lewes, East Sussex BN7 2NZ

Creative Director: Peter Bridgewater
Designer: John Grain
Editorial Director: Sophie Collins
Managing Editor: Anne Townley
Editor: Viv Croot
Studio Photography: Guy Ryecart
Picture Researcher: Lynda Marshall

Printed in China

This book is typeset in Caslon and Gill

Note: The treatment options offered in this book
should be considered as reference sources only.
They are not intended to substitute for a qualified
medical practitioner's diagnosis, advice, treatment
and prescribed medication. Always consult a qualified
practitioner for proper medical care.

Contents

Introduction

Modern medicine as we know it is only about 60 years old. Most of the complementary therapies, however, have stood the test of many centuries. In order to understand the current interest in complementary approaches, it is perhaps important that we acknowledge both the value and the shortcomings of modern medicine.

In the Western world, the accepted therapy is that practiced by allopathic physicians, those who have a doctorate in medicine. Allopathic medicine is founded on the clear-cut understanding of anatomy, physiology, and biochemistry. However, it was the introduction of antibiotics and tranquilizers in the 1940s that revolutionized the pharmacological approaches now so dominant in Western medicine. At the same time, technology improved our ability both to anesthetize patients and to perform very complex operative procedures. Nevertheless, it has been documented by both Dr. John Knowles, president of the Rockefeller Foundation, and Dr. Thomas McKeown, of Nuffield, England, that only 8 percent of the increased longevity that we have come to expect in the past 100 years is the result of modern medicine. The other 92 percent is due to better sanitation and nutrition. Furthermore, Dr. Knowles has emphasized that 85 percent of illnesses result from an unhealthy lifestyle: overeating, lack of exercise, excess alcohol consumption, smoking, and so on.

Dr. Hans Selye, scientist and physician, whose research proved so effectively the role of stress as the root of disease, demonstrated that stress can be the result of chemical, physical, or emotional pressures. The most common chemical stressors are tobacco, alcohol, sugar, and a wide variety of toxins in our environment. The most common physical stressors are inactivity and trauma. Emotional stress is generally the result of interpersonal conflicts. To these basic stressors, we now must add electromagnetic contamination, which can clearly affect our health, and radiation. Both of these influences have multiplied dramatically in the past century.

As early as the 1920s Dr. Edmund Jacobson demonstrated that 80 percent of a wide variety of illnesses could be controlled with such simple techniques as progressive relaxation. At the same time, Dr. J.H. Schultz in Germany showed that 80 percent of stress illnesses could be addressed with autogenic training, a form of self-hypnosis. Scientists who have studied the benefits of modern medicine now recognize that drugs and surgery are primarily useful in acute illnesses where they may be lifesaving. But in many chronic illnesses, the field of complementary therapy offers a safer and more effective approach.

Acupuncture, used for at least 4,000 years in the East found its way into the West through the explorations of Marco Polo and acupuncture has been used in France for at least 300 years. It was widely used in the United States in the 19th century only to disappear with the advent of 20th-century scientific medicine. It is now known that acupuncture can restore fertility in two thirds of infertile men, an accomplishment which cannot be equaled with modern scientific medicine. Migraines and most pain problems can be better treated with acupuncture than with drugs or surgery.

Relaxation in all of its forms is one of the great antidotes to stress. Jacobson, early in this century, was the first to demonstrate the physiological balancing aspects of deep relaxation. More recently, Benson of Harvard has shown that 20 minutes of deep relaxation twice a day lowers insulin requirements and epinephrine production by 50 percent for the entire 24-hour period. The only antidote that comes close as a stress modulator is physical exercise.

Homeopathy, introduced at a time when allopathic medicine was probably more dangerous than helpful, has been demonstrated to be as effective for treating osteoarthritic pain as acetaminophen, the drug doctors prescribe most. There is also excellent scientific support for its use in rheumatoid arthritis and increasingly in other illnesses.

Aromatherapy affects the limbic system, the center of our emotions, and recent scientific studies have demonstrated that aromatherapy can be effective in alopecia aerate, for which there is no good pharmaceutical approach.

Herbal medicine is actually the foundation of modern pharmacology. Each year new extracts of herbs are developed into specific drugs but traditional herbal therapy remains the standard in much of the Eastern world and has a great deal to offer those of us in the West.

Dr. Lushka long ago demonstrated the scientific value of color as a psychodiagnostic tool and color is one of the prime influences on that central emotional regulating center, the limbic system.

Yoga, Tai Chi, and dance therapy all offer cardiovascular benefits, stress reduction, and mental/emotional balancing techniques. And, of course, these therapies offer the additional potential benefits associated with meditation since they are all forms of movement meditation.

Naturopathy blends many of the natural approaches briefly mentioned here and most particularly emphasizes good nutrition. Prior to 1940, the vast majority of people ate food that was raised within 50 miles of their homes. Now throughout at least most of the Western world, the vast majority of food is not only grown hundreds of thousands of miles away from its consumption, but huge amounts of it have been highly processed and often deprived of their greatest health-giving nutrients.

At the beginning of the 20th century, a major revolution took place in modern scientific medicine. At the beginning of the 21st century, the revolution that is spreading throughout the world is a return to more traditional complementary therapy. As Sir William Osler stated over 100 years ago, "Far more important than what the physician does is the patient's belief and the physician's belief in what the physician does." Your belief, your attitude, your self-responsibility for choosing a healthy lifestyle, and selecting the appropriate

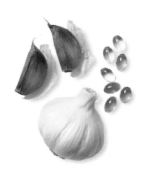

complementary approaches to health are the foundation for 21st-century medicine.

C. Norman Shealy, M.D. Ph.D.
Founder, Shealy Institute for Comprehensive Health Care, Founding President, American Holistic Medical Association

LIFESTYLE
THERAPIES

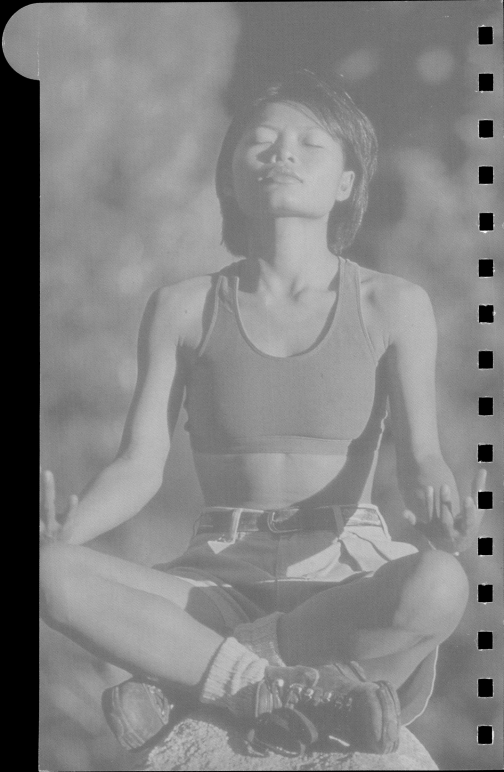

Naturopathy, relaxation, visualization, and meditation are probably the best way into the world of complementary therapies for the newcomer. They are the lifestyle therapies, designed to bring you to the peak of your personal well-being in body, mind, and soul. They address what you eat (naturopathy), how you deal with stress (relaxation), how you keep mental equilibrium (visualization), and how you maintain self-awareness (meditation). Easy to do, they are suitable for anyone of any age and in any physical condition, and can be practiced at home with no special equipment. A practitioner is advised to help you get started, but many of the principles of these therapies can be easily applied by individuals.

Naturopathy

Naturopathy is considered to be "original medicine," and is the earliest form of medical treatment in the Western world, having its foundation in the teachings of the Ancient Greek physician, Hippocrates. He prescribed diet, massage, hydrotherapy, and psychosomatics, which form the core of naturopathy today. The basic tenet that only nature heals is the essence of naturopathic philosophy. The practitioner attempts to help the patient to eliminate disease through improving general health, rather than specifically aiming at the clinical problem. When the individual's overall health is raised, disease cannot exist. In naturopathy prevention is as much a focus as cure.

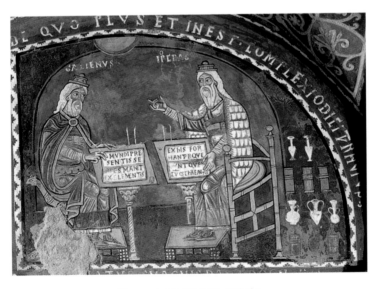

Hippocrates (c.460–c.370 BCE), the Greek physician, was well known throughout Greece and Asia Minor and founded the Hippocratic school of medicine, which greatly influenced Western medical science until the 18th century.

WILL IT HELP?

- Naturopathy is a way of life as much as a treatment form and is not a quick fix. It encourages an individual to be responsible for his or her own long-term health and gives the information to make this possible.
- However, since naturopathy treats the whole person and aims to raise overall health it is beneficial in a wide range of clinical problems, including infective and degenerative conditions.
- Naturopathy offers a lifestyle which focuses on preventing disease by encouraging a positive state of health and maintaining a good health profile.

 ## BENEFITS

- A great advantage of naturopathy is that it has virtually no dangerous side effects, since it concentrates on beneficial changes of lifestyle, including diet changes, exercise, and discouraging harmful life habits such as smoking.
- The changes encouraged by the naturopath are designed to be effective over the long term and tend by definition to be gentle in approach.
- Through involving the health and physiological efficiency of the individual, all systems potentially benefit.

 ## CAUTION

- In certain cases, such as with diabetes, diet changes must be monitored by a registered practitioner.
- Exercise prescription, hydrotherapy, and fasting should always be supervised by an experienced practitioner.
- Patients suffering from Raynaud's disease should use hydrotherapy only under practitioner advice.

Traditional naturopathy

The focus of naturopathic practice is on the maintenance of health rather than the cure of disease and its philosophy is that the body has the ability to heal itself provided it is given the correct support. The mechanisms of health maintenance within this form of therapy include nutrition and dietetics, fasting, massage, hydrotherapy, lifestyle manipulation, and psychology or counseling.

Some naturopaths insist that other forms of complementary or alternative medicine, such as acupuncture, homeopathy, and herbal medicine, should be included under the naturopathic umbrella. The traditional naturopath, however, does not see naturopathy as encompassing these forms of therapy, but believes that they stand in their own right. While each is compatible with naturopathy they are all separate and distinct practices and do not form part of it. An awareness and recognition of, and indeed respect for, these other forms of therapy is nevertheless considered to be very important.

A thorough understanding of medical science is a fundamental part of the knowledge base required for naturopathic practice and the student

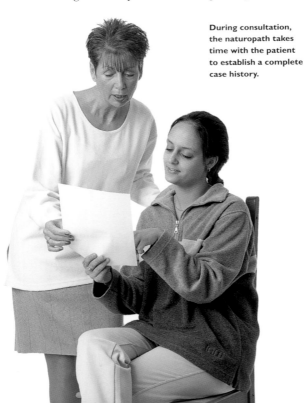

During consultation, the naturopath takes time with the patient to establish a complete case history.

naturopath studies the basic medical sciences of anatomy, physiology, pathology, and diagnosis which form the foundation of applied clinical practice. In naturopathy the major focus of clinical treatment is dietetics and fasting, soft tissue manipulation (massage), hydrotherapy, immunology, and counseling. To train as a naturopath usually takes four years of full-time study, leading to a BSc degree.

SEVEN DAY DIET RECORD SHEET

MONDAY

Breakfast 6.00AM – 10.00AM	Lunch 10.00AM – 4.00PM	Dinner 4.00PM – 11.00PM
BREAKFAST 7.30 Bowl of cornflakes with milk 2 pieces of toast (brown bread) cup of coffee 11 O'CLOCK cup of coffee chocolate bar	LUNCH 10'CLOCK tuna and mayonnaise sandwich piece of fruit cake glass of apple juice 3.30 cup of tea	6.00 cup of tea slice of bread and butter DINNER 8 O'CLOCK 2 lamb chops potatoes (1 cup) carrots (½ cup) glass of water

As part of the initial consultation, the naturopath will need to get a full picture of your diet, so a detailed record of what you have eaten over the previous week is essential.

UNDERGOING TREATMENT   In a consultation with a naturopath the patient will be asked for a complete case history, including a full personal health record, a brief family health record, and a detailed description of what is wrong. Some time will be devoted to taking an outline dietary history and personal profile, including stress analysis. A physical examination follows, with a routine screen of blood pressure, heart rate, heart and lung sounds, reflexes, and palpation of the abdomen, as appropriate to the presenting condition. The naturopath then discusses the findings with the patient and a treatment regime is devised. Depending on the presenting condition some massage may be given to aid stress relief or, for example, to affect the abdominal organs of the digestive tract. The treatment program will include advice on diet, exercise prescription, counseling, and advice regarding hydrotherapy as appropriate.

The patient will usually then be requested to compile a detailed account of his or her diet over the next seven days before coming for a further consultation. This seven-day diet record is very important and it notes exactly what is eaten, when, and broadly how much. The patient keeps an ongoing record, and since the report does not rely on memory it gives a clearer and more accurate base from which the naturopath can assess and realign the diet if necessary.

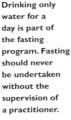

FASTING AND EXERCISE   Fasting is often recommended by the naturopath. This should never be attempted without full practitioner support and advice, since it could be dangerous if followed without experienced support. Properly controlled, however, it is a useful and powerful method of encouraging healing. Fasting plays a part in the observation of many philosophies and religions around the world and there is a wide experience of its use, although few people in the Western world now resort to this tried and tested practice. The naturopath will usually incorporate fasting with an uninitiated patient slowly, generally starting with a half-day mono-diet of grapes. On this diet the patient has a light breakfast, followed by grapes and grape juice for the rest of the day until evening, and then a light salad. This gently exposes him or her to the concept of reduced dietary intake and gives confidence in the technique. The process is slowly expanded until the patient is prepared and confident enough to embark on a three- or five-day regime. A three-day regime involves a restricted, light diet on day one; water only on day two; and a return to a light diet on day three, with a

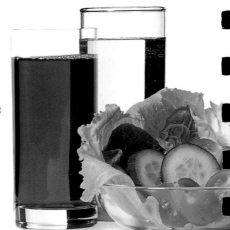

Drinking only
water for a
day is part of
the fasting
program. Fasting
should never
be undertaken
without the
supervision of
a practitioner.

return to a light normal diet on day four. The five-day regime has the same outline program except that days two and three are on water only. The fasting process should ideally be performed on rest days—usually at the weekend. The object of the fast is to give a rest to the system.

If exercise prescription is given it will usually start in a similar way to a fast, with small incremental changes to one's life pattern, beginning by increased walking, and rising to more specific and taxing exercise as appropriate to the patient.

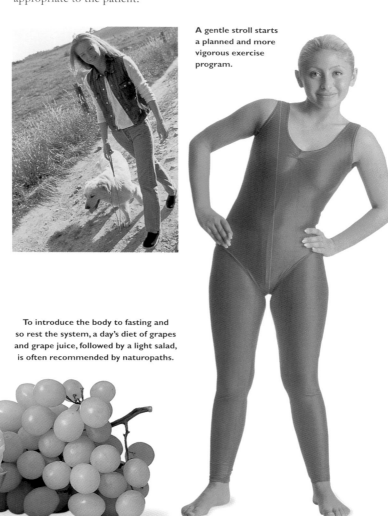

A gentle stroll starts a planned and more vigorous exercise program.

To introduce the body to fasting and so rest the system, a day's diet of grapes and grape juice, followed by a light salad, is often recommended by naturopaths.

HYDROTHERAPY Hydrotherapy involves the use of water, which may be in the form of showers, packs, or baths and may be cold or hot, or the two alternating. The patient is taken slowly through incremental changes in order to become competent in the technique and to experience changes over time. The cold shower is often used to encourage an improvement in blood supply to the area treated. Water is used straight from the cold faucet, usually for a short time (15–20 seconds) and this results in a reflex increase in local blood supply. Paradoxically patients suffering from cold hands or feet or "restless leg syndrome" can benefit from this technique practiced routinely each morning. The use of alternating hot and cold water is often employed for inflammatory conditions.

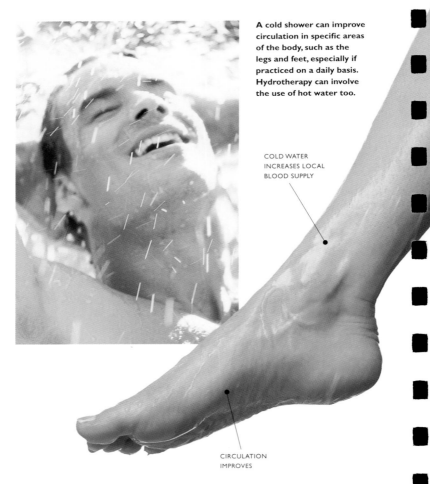

A cold shower can improve circulation in specific areas of the body, such as the legs and feet, especially if practiced on a daily basis. Hydrotherapy can involve the use of hot water too.

COLD WATER
INCREASES LOCAL
BLOOD SUPPLY

CIRCULATION
IMPROVES

COUNSELING   The counseling element of the naturopath's work involves attempting to address issues of an emotional or psychological nature to bring an awareness and understanding of such problems to the patient. Naturopaths are neither psychoanalysts nor psychiatrists, and their area of expertise extends only to guiding the patient's awareness of psychosomatic factors. The naturopath recognizes the influence of psychological issues in diseased states as being of profound importance, as well as being fundamental to the healing process. The general approach of the naturopath will be to integrate all the advice and treatment into a complete entity so that the counseling element is woven into the consultation process.

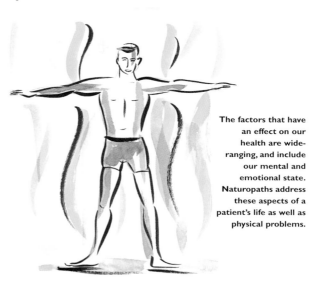

The factors that have an effect on our health are wide-ranging, and include our mental and emotional state. Naturopaths address these aspects of a patient's life as well as physical problems.

 Is naturopathy compatible with conventional medicine?
Naturopathy can be practiced alongside conventional or allopathic medicine. However, because of the broad difference in approach, careful monitoring and explanation of principle to the patient may be necessary.

 Is a practitioner necessary?
If a patient is suffering from a specific condition or disease, then a qualified naturopathic practitioner is essential for clinical judgments. However, self-help may be appropriate if the individual has a competent level of knowledge.

Relaxation therapies

It is now generally accepted that numerous medical conditions, such as colds and influenza, migraines, asthma, stomach ulcers, irritable bowel syndrome, colitis, neck and back problems, eczema, heart attacks and strokes, hypertension, anxiety, depression, insomnia, even cancer, and AIDS, are either triggered off or exacerbated by stress and repressed or unresolved emotional issues. However, what is not widely appreciated is that, in addition to contributing to. many illnesses, stress in its broadest context is one of the most potent disrupters of the harmonious relationship between the body, the mind, and the immune system, the proper functioning of which is essential for keeping us healthy and which prevents susceptibility to disease.

As stress and unresolved emotions are such important factors in affecting our health, there have been many techniques developed over the years to try and enable individuals to manage their stress levels and thus combat its detrimental effects. Some are of course much more effective than others, and individuals have to try different techniques until they find the one that suits them and their personality. Autogenic Training is one of the most effective methods of stress management that I have come across over the last 20 years, and is the focus of this chapter.

Stress is a major contributor to ill health, with stress in the workplace being one of today's principal hazards. Relaxation techniques can help to manage stress levels.

What is Autogenic Training?

Autogenic Training is probably one of the most effective, powerful, yet simple techniques of relaxation, self-empowerment, and self-healing that has been developed in the West. It was first developed by the neuro-psychologist Dr. J.H. Schultze in Germany in the early 1930s, and later perfected by Dr. W. Luthe. It consists of a series of simple mental exercises designed to turn off the stressful "fight-or-flight" mechanism in the body and turn on the restorative and recuperative rhythms associated with profound psychophysical relaxation. It has been scientifically shown that this method, when practiced daily, brings about results on the mental level comparable to those achieved by Eastern forms of meditation, and on the physical level produces the chemical and physiological body changes associated with those who train hard for physical or athletic activities. It also enables trainees to get in touch with their deeper feelings of repressed emotions, if that is relevant and appropriate, and deal with them effectively through specific additional, practical off-loading exercises, so that the deep states of peace and tranquillity that are achieved can be maintained on a prolonged basis.

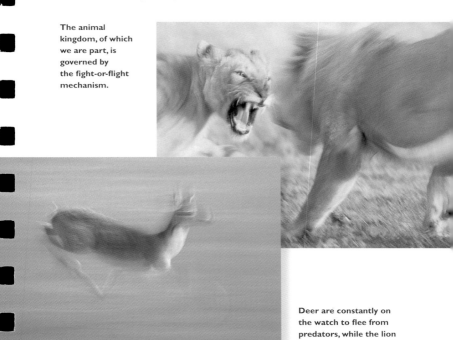

The animal kingdom, of which we are part, is governed by the fight-or-flight mechanism.

Deer are constantly on the watch to flee from predators, while the lion will turn and fight.

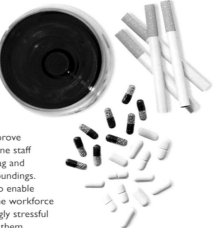

WILL IT HELP?

• Autogenic Training is a
key preventive measure.
   • It can be used to help you
take control of your life as
an aid in giving up smoking,
coming off tranquillizers
and sleeping pills, and losing
excess weight.
     • It can help athletes to improve
their performance and airline staff
to fight the effects of jet lag and
insomnia in strange surroundings.
      • It is used in industry to enable
the management and the workforce
to cope with increasingly stressful
demands imposed on them.

**Numerous
athletes use
Autogenic
Training to
focus on goals
and improve
performance.**

**Autogenic Training can
help you to cut the stressors
of smoking, tranquillizers,
and alcohol out of your life.**

 ### BENEFITS

• Autogenic Training helps to restore
the harmony between mind, body, and
immune system and thus helps to deal
effectively with psychosomatic illnesses
and their manifestations.
   • It helps to harmonize the interrelated
activities between the two halves of the
brain and thus mobilize latent creative
talents. It also improves concentration
and coordination.
     • Most importantly, it enables individuals to
get into the space of peace and relaxation
deep within themselves where all the self-
healing, self-regulatory, and self-normalizing
processes take place.

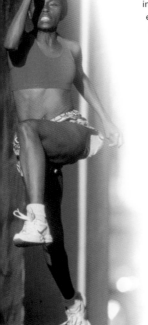

 ### CAUTION

• No one suffering from epilepsy, insulin-
dependent diabetes, psychotic depression,
or schizophrenia should undertake Autogenic
Training without first consulting a qualified
practitioner.

Self-healing

Autogenic Training is particularly appealing to the modern Western mind, because, unlike many forms of meditation and yoga, it has no cultural, religious, or cosmological overtones, and requires no special clothing or unusual postures or positions. But perhaps most importantly of all, as the name implies, physical and mental relaxation, as well as feelings of peace and tranquillity, are generated from within oneself and are not dependent on any external values, philosophies, or therapists. Furthermore, it is a functional tool that can be used anywhere and at any time, unlike certain other forms of relaxation technique. The deep space of stillness with which the user gets in touch can also be utilized for self-healing and empowerment, especially in conjunction with visualization and positive affirmations.

Autogenic Training is used in many Western countries to help pregnant women cope with the demands on their body.

This technique, very popular in the 1970s and early 1980s, involves the use of electronic instruments in order to gauge the ability of the participant to use his or her conscious mind and active concentration to try to alter physiological functions of the body, such as pulse rate and blood pressure. Information about the physical state is constantly fed back, via instruments, to the participant so that he or she can modify the breathing or muscle tension to achieve the desired result. This goal-oriented program can actually serve to increase stress in some individuals; if they are unable to achieve the physiological changes as measured by the instruments, their feelings of inadequacy may be reinforced. This, together with the cost of the gadgets and the development of other effective techniques, has caused the loss of interest in this technique in the UK. It has now been largely superseded by other relaxation techniques that do not involve the use of active concentration and instruments.

BIOFEEDBACK

How it's done

Autogenic Training involves the use of a series of mental exercises designed to teach the trainee to concentrate on normal and natural physical sensations, such as heaviness and warmth, in various parts of the body, and by so doing, learn to bypass conscious processes and proceed to a state of deep relaxation. The focus of attention progresses from the limbs to the heart and circulation, the breathing and the nervous system, and thus to deep within oneself. The trainee learns to control the hormones and chemicals that are released via the intervention of the nervous system and that lead toward the enhancement of his or her health and state of well-being. The ability to do this and achieve "passive concentration" at will breaks through the vicious cycle of excessive stress and tension, irrespective of its origin, and enables the individual to use the technique at any time to deal with any stressful situation or event.

FLOTATION THERAPY

The technique was first devised by Dr. Lilley, a neurophysiologist, in 1950 and was later perfected, with many modifications, in the United States. It involves the use of an egg-shaped, light-blue fiberglass tank, about as wide as a double bed, with 15in (37.5cm) of water at the bottom. High buoyancy is achieved by dissolving a large amount of Epsom salts in the water, which is kept at 93°F (33.9°C), normal skin temperature, as is the air temperature. The participant, usually nude but possibly in a swimming costume, lies in the tank in a totally darkened, silent setting, thereby subject to minimal sensory stimulation. Although it can be quite relaxing for some people, others can become disoriented and feel as if they are turning in a whirlpool or even overturning. Most importantly, it can create a sense of claustrophobia, anxiety, and panic in susceptible individuals, despite claims to the contrary. Its other disadvantages are expense, time—each session is between 60 and 90 minutes—and the lack of well-equipped centers run by properly trained staff.

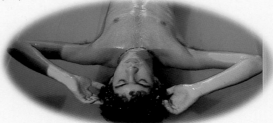

**The flotation tank is designed to create
minimal sensory perception to promote relaxation
and concentration, but does not suit everyone.**

Autogenic advantages

1   Simple, effective, powerful
2   Can be used anywhere and at any time
3   Self-generated
4   Passive concentration takes away the fear and anxiety of "Am I doing it right?"
5   Helps with self-healing
6   The longer it is used, the more effective it becomes
7   Powerful preventive measure
8   Enables safe release of emotions
9   Clears backlog of stress
10   Revitalizes and rejuvenates
11   Enhances creativity and positive attributes
12   Improves performance in sport, education, aviation, business, and industry
13   No religious or cosmological connotations

 Is Autogenic Training compatible with conventional medicine?
It can be safely combined with all known forms of conventional and complementary therapies to enhance their effectiveness.

Is a practitioner necessary?
A trainer is not essential since the technique can be learned from the book *Autogenic Training* by Dr. Kai Kermani, provided the precautions and instructions are followed carefully. The personal touch of a trainer may benefit some trainees, particularly regarding initial motivation to do the mental exercises regularly.

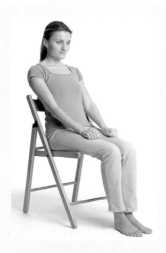

Clenching and unclenching the muscles is a user-friendly form of self-help relaxation.

JACOBSEN'S PROGRESSIVE MUSCULAR RELAXATION

This simple technique can be used by anyone at any time, especially when tension is felt in the muscles. It can be used before any other relaxation technique if muscular tension is a particular problem. It involves breathing deeply and slowly in and out while gently clenching and unclenching different muscle groups, starting from the toes and feet, moving up through the calves, thighs, buttocks, abdomen, back, neck, upper arms, elbows and hands, and ending with the muscles of the face. The process can be repeated, until the tightness in the muscles is released.

Visualization

Visualization, the use of the imagination for healing purposes, is one of the oldest of all known therapies. One of its earliest recorded uses was as early as 1000 BCE, by Aesclepius, a Greek physician, healer, and philosopher. It was because of the effectiveness and success of the therapies he advocated that, following his death, a series of "healing temples" called Aesclepia were set up in Greece, Italy, and Turkey. These were the true forerunners of present-day holistic medical centers only now being set up in the US. In the Western world, visualization lost its popularity with the rise of scientific, conventional medicine some 200 years ago but it continued to be practiced by shamans (folk-medicine healers) in other parts of the world. The effectiveness of this therapy is now being recognized once more and it has begun to be used by both physicians and psychologists.

Aesclepius showed the Ancient Greeks that the mind was a powerful healer, and founded healing centers to promote this therapy. Today there is a resurgence of interest in visualization, both for healing and self-improvement.

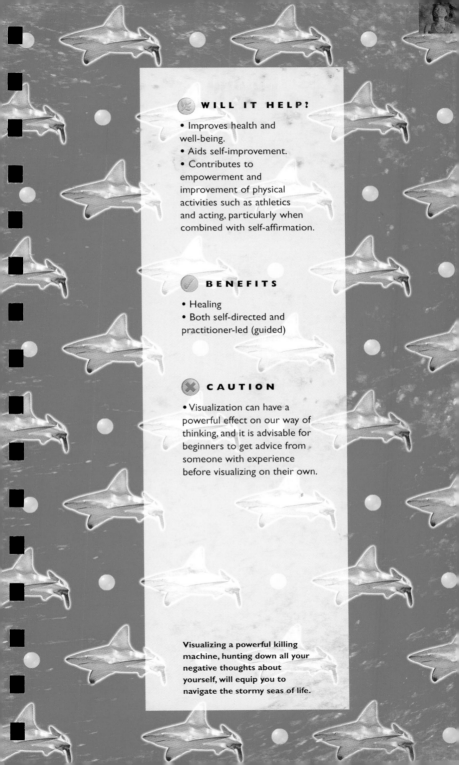

WILL IT HELP?

- Improves health and well-being.
- Aids self-improvement.
- Contributes to empowerment and improvement of physical activities such as athletics and acting, particularly when combined with self-affirmation.

BENEFITS

- Healing
- Both self-directed and practitioner-led (guided)

CAUTION

- Visualization can have a powerful effect on our way of thinking, and it is advisable for beginners to get advice from someone with experience before visualizing on their own.

Visualizing a powerful killing machine, hunting down all your negative thoughts about yourself, will equip you to navigate the stormy seas of life.

The power of the image

Visualization therapy, also known as imagery or image work, is based on the belief that by thinking we can create images which we can use negatively or positively. By learning to control our imaginations, we control our thoughts; control our thoughts and we control our emotions; control our emotions and we clear our minds for higher levels of thought. At these times we can gain insights that we never thought possible and consequently mature in our perceptions and emotional response.

We cannot escape being a product of our own thoughts and imagination. We spend more time in our imaginations than most people realize. In the negative aspect, we may spend time misinterpreting, jumping to conclusions, indulging in unfulfilled desires, resenting circumstances, misjudging others and ourselves; in the positive aspect, we plan, hope, dream, fantasize, perceive, and use our creative intelligence. Reality sets the stage, but the imagination creates what we believe is the plot behind the scene.

NEUTRALIZING THE NEGATIVE A powerful charge is given to images when they have an emotional content, especially if fear or pain are involved. When a stressful response to the world focuses our imagination on the negative aspects of our environment, we become the creators of a negative reality. Negative emotions blind us to many productive options that are available. The point is not to be tricked into trusting and accepting anything that we perceive while in a negative state of mind. If we learn to look through the glasses of love, faith, hope, patience, forgiveness, reverence, and charity, we will see life in an undistorted and compassionate way. It is up to us whether we decide to spend a lifetime in the world of negative imagery or take a bold and courageous step into a state of positive and creative imagination in our thoughts and hearts.

Self-directed visualization

Self-directed visualization can be used in a number of different ways and for different purposes. If it is to be used for self-healing, then the individual relaxes and once in that space of deep relaxation concentrates on where the problem might be and allows spontaneous healing images to come up. It may take a few sessions before something happens.

Once a healing image has come up, the client continues using that image until the problem is resolved or something else comes up. For instance, one particular client whose retina was being destroyed as a result of disease had a spontaneous image that the scar tissues were bubbling up and disappearing into the fluid of the eye like the bubbles of champagne

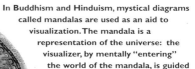

In Buddhism and Hinduism, mystical diagrams called mandalas are used as an aid to visualization. The mandala is a representation of the universe: the visualizer, by mentally "entering" the world of the mandala, is guided through the cosmic processes of disintegration and reintegration.

in a glass, with resultant improvement in his condition. While you wait for a spontaneous image to come up, you can work with one of the established images described in many books; for instance, little sharks eating up cancer cells. The beneficial effects of visualization can further be enhanced by the addition of positive affirmations.

The technique of imagery can also be used for releasing emotions or unnecessary and unwanted attachment to people, places, and situations in one's life, and for improving performance in an athletic context.

Practitioner-led or guided visualization

The technique used to induce relaxation and altered state of consciousness is dependent on the practitioners' preferences. Common techniques are meditation, hypnosis, and Autogenic Training. Visualization can either be done in a group setting or individually, when more specific issues can be tackled. The main aim of the technique is the manipulation of the client's mental imaging from a negative to a positive state in order to support healing. This could be for recovery from disease or disability or improving confidence and feelings of self-worth. Some therapists use guided visualization to take a person back to their childhood to try and elucidate what is contributing to their current problems. This regression can even involve a past life in a previous incarnation because issues from that time can have a detrimental effect on our health in this life.

Is visualization compatible with conventional medicine?
The effectiveness of conventional treatments can be enhanced by visualization, which creates a positive and receptive state of mind.

Is a practitioner necessary?
No, but it is preferable to get advice before visualizing on your own.

Meditation

Meditation—a practice that encourages deep relaxation and self-awareness—is common in the East, where it is an integral part of a number of religious practices, including Hinduism and Buddhism. However, some of the more modern innovators such as those involved with the Transcendental Meditation movement (which is based on the Indian Vedanta religious philosophy known as the Science of Creative Intelligence) have tried to shake off meditation's religious connotations and make it more appropriate as a therapy for Western lifestyles.

Maharishi Mahesh Yogi, the founder of Transcendental Meditation.

Transcendental Meditation

Transcendental Meditation (TM), founded in the 1940s by the Maharishi Mahesh Yogi, became popular in the West in the 1960s. TM is based more on specific meditation techniques than on religious or philosophical beliefs. The Maharishi developed a simple form of meditation that could be practiced easily in the modern world. TM uses various Sanskrit mantras, each of which is a word or phrase. When the mantra is repeated in the mind over a period of time, it helps the user to quieten and still his or her thought activity and find a deeper level of consciousness. It is claimed that the practitioner finds deep relaxation, which leads to improved health and enhanced inner joy, vitality, and creativity.

To practice TM, a person must be initiated by a teacher. This involves sessions of formal instruction, followed by a ceremony in which the applicant makes offerings and receives his or her mantra, selected by the teacher on the basis of temperament and occupation. In three or four subsequent "checking" sessions the person meditates under the teacher's observation; the meditator then begins meditating independently twice a day for periods of 20 minutes each. Further levels of training are available.

WILL IT HELP?

• Meditation has been shown to reduce high blood pressure and to help alleviate insomnia. It also encourages greater physical and mental vitality, and is said to reverse the visible effects of aging.

 BENEFITS

• Reduces stress and insomnia.
• Increases happiness, intelligence, creativity, and energy.
• Improves memory, health, and relationships.
• Reduces high blood pressure.
• Reverses the visible effects of aging.
• Increases physical and mental vitality.

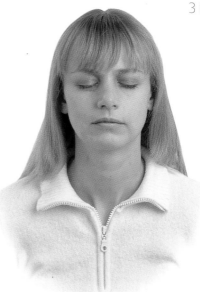

You can either practice Transcendental Meditation alone or join with other people for group meditation.

 CAUTION

• The use of a teacher is essential.
• Meditation can lose its effectiveness if an individual gets in touch with deep emotional issues, because nothing within meditation teaches ways of dealing with these.

Burmese monks follow a Buddhist tradition that stipulates severe discipline in order to achieve self-liberation.

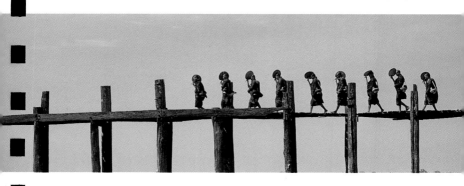

Buddhist meditation

People who undertake Buddhist meditation often also adopt the principles of Buddhist life, though this is by no means essential. Broadly speaking, there are two basic forms of Buddhist meditation. Both are powerful and have been practiced in various forms and combinations.

YOGIC MEDITATION The first type of Buddhist meditation, which was emphasized in the classical Buddhist texts, is closely related to a Hindu tradition of yoga practice. It involves concentrating on moral, intellectual, or abstract issues, which in time will lead to spiritual purification. This initial state is usually attained in four stages.

1 In the first stage, the meditator achieves detachment from sensual desires and impure states of mind through analysis and reflection and thereby attains an emotional state of satisfaction and joy.

2 In the second stage, intellectual activities are relinquished to a complete inner serenity, the mind being in a state of "one-pointedness," or total concentration.

3 In the third stage, every emotion, including joy, disappears, leaving the meditator indifferent to everything, while remaining completely conscious.

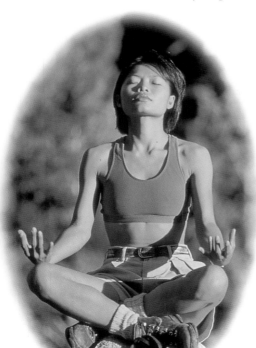

4 The fourth stage is abandonment of any sense of satisfaction, pain, or serenity, because any inclination to a good or bad state of mind has disappeared. The meditator thus enters a state of supreme purity and pure consciousness.

Buddhist meditation has grown in popularity. It is based on the teachings of the Buddha, Gautama Siddhartha (c.563–c.483 BCE), an Indian prince who renounced his life of luxury to seek solutions to the suffering and transience of the human condition.

INSIGHT MEDITATION The second form of Buddhist meditation is called "insight" meditation. In recent times this form, which was also mentioned in classical Buddhist texts, has received greater emphasis, presumably because it is easier for the modern meditator to undertake, especially in the Western world.

Insight meditation involves concentrating on more concrete situations or objects—breathing, the flame of a lighted candle, or a flower. In the case of the latter two objects, the person meditating initially keeps his or her eyes open, closing them once "one-pointedness" of vision is achieved. This is the point when the double or multiple images seen during concentration disappear, leaving a single image. Once this has happened, the meditator closes his or her eyes and allows the mind to wander.

The meditation period can last from a few minutes to as long as the meditator wishes. The act of deliberate and intense concentration leads to one-pointedness of the mind, which in turn is used to attain insight into the Buddhist truth that all reality is without self and is impermanent. From the Buddhist perspective, such insight may enable progress to total spiritual enlightenment, or nirvana.

By concentrating on an object, such as a flower or a candle flame, the meditator achieves one-pointedness of the mind.

The haunting chants that emerged from the medieval monasteries are still enjoyed today as a musical form or for more spiritual purposes. Chanting has reemerged as a way of moving into a meditative state.

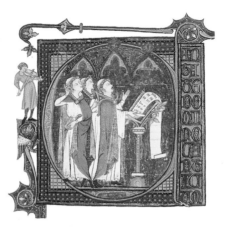

CHANT

This is the general name for unaccompanied vocal liturgical music, which often leads the participant to an altered state of consciousness. It can refer to melodies of the Orthodox, Roman Catholic, and Anglican branches of Christianity but is also prevalent in other traditions, such as Buddhism and Hinduism. The texts of Anglican chants are usually from the Book of Common Prayer. Other well-known forms of chant are Byzantine and Gregorian. The participant can either listen to these chants sung by others or participate in the process of harmonizing.

In Buddhist and Sai Baba chanting, the participant repeats aloud and repeatedly a word or phrase, often in Sanskrit, so that it has no emotional or intellectual connotations. As a consequence, the person chanting will pass into a meditative state of altered consciousness.

One of the most useful forms of individual chanting is making the specific sounds of the seven main chakras (energy centers). These are: "o," the deepest and lowest in pitch and tonality (the position of this chakra is in the soft part between the anus and vulva/scrotum); "ou" (just below the navel); "ah" (solar plexus); "ai" (heart); "ee" (throat) ; "om," with concentration on the "m" (center of forehead); and "ng," such as in the word "sing," being the highest pitched (situated in the crown region). Regular daily chanting of these chakra sounds helps to clear a person's energy centers and field, helping to energize and refresh the individual.

Is meditation compatible with conventional medicine?
Meditation creates a positive outlook, which aids conventional medicine.

Is a practitioner necessary?
It is essential that meditation is introduced by a qualified teacher.

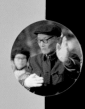

FEELGOOD THERAPIES

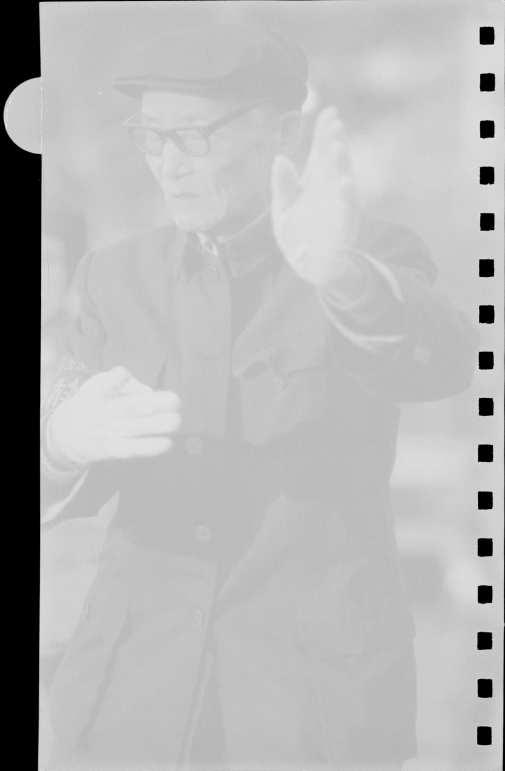

One Western and two Eastern therapies offer a choice of paths to physical confidence and body awareness. The Alexander Technique, Tai Chi, and Chi Kung offer people of all ages and minimum physical fitness the chance to feel in tune with, and in control of, their bodies. For Western readers, the Alexander Technique may be initially easier to understand since it is based on familiar concepts such as posture and deportment. However, the proliferation of Tai Chi and Chi Kung classes in the West indicates that the Eastern therapies, based on balance, harmony, and maximum impact with minimum physical effort, are becoming very popular.

All three therapies require a practitioner and some classes, but can be practiced individually once the techniques have been learned.

Alexander Technique

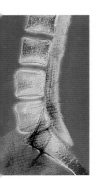

Developed in the 1890s by the Australian Frederick Matthias Alexander to overcome his own vocal and breathing problems, the Alexander Technique is now one of the most widely known and used complementary disciplines, providing therapeutic benefits through reeducation and empowerment for self-help. By observing himself in the way he stood and moved, and the unnecessary movements and tension that occurred when preparing to carry out an action, Alexander realized that the way we "use ourselves" affects how well we function. Thus was born a technique in which awareness of mind and body, and how they work together, may be used to overcome certain ailments and improve performance.

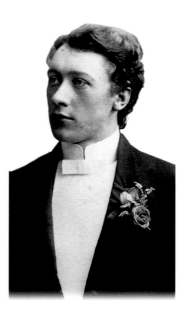

Frederick Matthias Alexander (1869–1955): "Every man, woman, and child holds within the possibility of physical perfection."

In this colored x-ray of the lumbar (lower) region of a human spine the vertebrae are seen as a line of green and yellow squares. To the right of them, shown in yellow, is the spinal cord.

WILL IT HELP?

• Lessons in the Alexander Technique will teach you a more natural way of moving and of supporting your weight, and a way of monitoring how you do this.

• The Alexander Technique is not a direct treatment or cure for specific illnesses and complaints. Instead, it is an educational method concerning what we can do to improve our overall functioning.

• In doing so, it may remove the root cause of many complaints when these are induced by our own habits. It also makes any activity we perform easier and more enjoyable.

 BENEFITS

• Improvement in balance and coordination, greater self-awareness, better presence, improved vocal function, reduced tension.

• May alleviate chronic back pain or other joint, muscle, or connective tissue problems, postural distortion, and digestive and breathing difficulties.

• Though not a psychotherapy or cure for psychological complaints, the Alexander Technique can bring some psychological benefits, such as greater self-confidence, reduced anxiety, and an enhanced ability to cope with stress.

 CAUTION

• The Alexander Technique cannot be learned properly without the presence and guidance of a qualified teacher.

• In order to gain lasting benefits, Alexander pupils should participate in the learning process and apply what they have learned to their everyday life.

The onset of misuse

The Alexander Technique is popularly described as helping with posture and relaxation. Although "good posture" and "being relaxed" are generally not thought to go hand in hand, to many people's surprise the Technique does satisfy both these objectives, and many others, by examining and changing how we carry out acts in our daily lives.

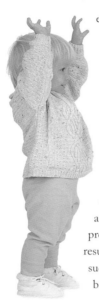

Young children, particularly at toddler age, are an example of exquisite poise. They move around freely, stand or sit easily with upright, yet relaxed and flowing backs, and perform their actions in a simple, direct way, using a suitable amount of effort. Their systems are functioning the way they are built to function, efficiently and as a whole. As we grow older, for any number of possible reasons, we develop harmful habits of excess tension and misguided effort. In the jargon of the Alexander Technique, we begin to "use ourselves" improperly. Since our overtense musculature is attached to our skeleton, it also pulls our posture out of alignment and generally compresses our structure. The excessive pressure or strain on various parts of the body that results from chronic poor use can lead to complaints such as back, neck, or shoulder pain, joint problems, breathing difficulties, and fatigue. It can also hamper our coordination and potential in many skilled activities such as athletics, singing, or playing a musical instrument.

Toddlers have excellent posture, they move freely and sit and stand with an upright back.

Habits of misuse become ingrained in our daily life and, like any habits, we perpetuate them without thinking about it. Usually we are not even aware of what we are doing. Fortunately, since misuse is something we do to ourselves unconsciously, the Alexander Technique shows us how to recognize and stop what we are doing, and how to consciously develop a way of supporting our weight and moving that is both natural and efficient, both relaxed and energized, like the child's. This often removes the root cause of a problem so that, in many cases, symptoms are subsequently alleviated. The pupil also experiences a sense of well-being, improved function, and better coordination in a variety of skills. The Technique has also been found useful for easier pregnancy and childbirth.

When we feel "right" or "wrong"

If we experience discomfort or pain, we suspect that something is "wrong," although we may not be able to tell what it is. It is tricky to notice and change our own imbalances of tension because they are with us all the time, so they feel normal. For instance, if you were to tense your stomach muscles on purpose, then you could easily relax them because you know they are contracting. Yet you may long have stopped feeling a tension that has become part of your everyday life. Take an extreme example: in a very stooped, tense person, a more upright, balanced stance often feels like leaning backward, although a look in the mirror reveals that this is not the case. Alexander called this "faulty sensory appreciation," meaning that, with time, harmful habits cause us to have a distorted feeling of what we are doing with our bodies.

Many people confuse the idea of using their body well with simplistic "body mechanics." For instance, they will say that to lift heavy objects, you must bend your knees and hips while keeping your back straight, instead of curving from the waist. This is not exactly wrong; however, assuming set body positions is not enough to use the body well, and usually leads to rigidity rather than to any fundamental change to a person's misuse. (Some people who adopt the above method have been known to develop knee pains in the place of back pain!) The person's basic habits of ingrained tension throughout the body do not change, so the internal pressure and strain exerted by any type of physical effort are simply increased, no matter what kind of superficial position one adopts.

By helping a person to recognize and shed bad posture habits, while presenting an experience of a more balanced, easy way of using the body, an Alexander teacher can help to restore a more reliable sensory perception, and thus enable the person to manage his or her own self-use.

Standing poorly may be so ingrained that we have a false sense of our own posture.

OBSERVE YOUR HABITS

Do you notice yourself using excessive effort and tension when:

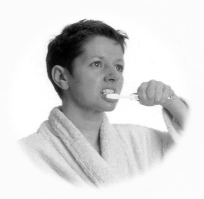

- Brushing your teeth?
- Doing the dishes?
- Driving a car?
- Riding a bicycle?
- Straining to run an extra half-mile?
- Working at a computer?

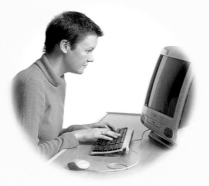

Do these activities also affect your posture, or cause discomfort or pain?

Can you imagine performing these activities with less tension?

If so, the Alexander Technique may be a suitable method for you to learn.

Learning the Alexander Technique

The Alexander Technique is taught in one-to-one lessons. Group courses can provide a general introduction, but do not give you enough personalized attention to become proficient in managing your use. During an Alexander lesson, you remain fully clothed, except for removing your shoes.

While looking at simple, everyday stances and movements, such as sitting on and rising from a chair, the Alexander teacher combines verbal instruction with manual guidance to your musculature. This guidance is not an outright manipulation, more like a gentle hand contact with subtle adjustments, especially around the neck, head,

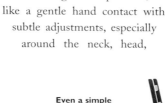

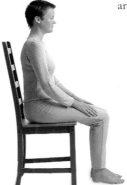

Even a simple movement, such as rising from a chair, can tell the Alexander teacher much about an individual's movement and poise and what steps need to be taken to rectify problems.

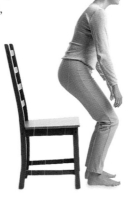

and back, giving you an experience of what the spoken instructions actually mean.

In so doing, the teacher helps to draw your attention to spots of excess tension, to consciously release those areas, and to gradually allow your entire structure to go from a state of compression and strain to a more natural length, width, and degree of muscle tone. The teacher's hands and your own mental volition cooperate to bring about change, and you will increasingly learn to direct this process by yourself. Postural distortions will gradually undo themselves as overtense muscles become more relaxed, overrelaxed ones become more toned, and movement becomes freer and lighter.

The number of Alexander lessons needed to achieve proficiency varies from person to person. As an average, most teachers recommend taking around 30 lessons at a minimum rate of once a week. Radical change comes about gradually, since we are dealing with the habits of a lifetime, but most people begin to experience benefits from the first few lessons.

LYING SEMISUPINE   Although you need a teacher to learn the Alexander Technique in its entirety, you might find the following procedure enjoyable and beneficial.

Lie on your back on a carpeted floor, with the back of your head resting supported on several inches of paperback books. Your neck should not be in contact with the books. Bend your knees, so that your feet are approximately 1–2ft (30–60cm) away from your buttocks, and roughly your shoulders' width apart. It is preferable to bend your elbows and rest your hands, palms down, on your stomach.

Allow the weight of your body to be supported by the floor—it is surprising how often we lie down yet still hold ourselves rigidly as if to keep ourselves up! Let your head rest comfortably on the books, allow your neck to soften and

HANDS, PALMS DOWN, ON STOMACH

A teacher may recommend the semi-supine position to help to release the pupil's muscles and joints.

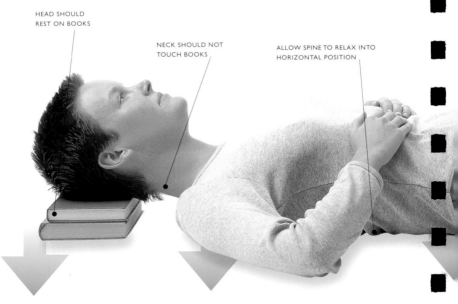

HEAD SHOULD REST ON BOOKS

NECK SHOULD NOT TOUCH BOOKS

ALLOW SPINE TO RELAX INTO HORIZONTAL POSITION

relax, and allow gravity to decompress and lengthen your spine in this horizontal position. Also think of allowing the shoulders to relax and the back to widen. Do not force anything, just allow your body to recover its natural shape, as your resting level of tension decreases.

If you lie this way for 15–20 minutes every day, you can begin to undo some of the rigidity and distortion caused by habits of misuse.

If you decide to take Alexander lessons, a teacher can demonstrate and explain additional principles for this procedure, and how to apply the Alexander Technique in standing and moving.

Is the Alexander Technique compatible with conventional medicine?
The Technique addresses underlying habits and may lessen the need for medical intervention for conditions related to posture.

Is a practitioner necessary?
You will need a teacher initially to learn the Technique.

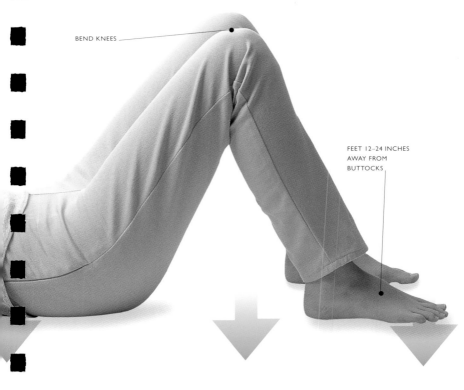

BEND KNEES

FEET 12–24 INCHES
AWAY FROM
BUTTOCKS

Tai Chi

"Tai Chi" is short for "tai chi chuan," and is the name given to a series of movements developed from a form of Chinese martial art created by Chang San Feng (1247–1368). The practice of the set Tai Chi forms is designed to bring about not only physical balance but also greater mental and emotional stability, and Tai Chi is now widely practiced for its great health benefits. The relaxed, flowing, circular movements are believed to encourage the flow of life-force energy known as "qi," or "chi," through the meridians, or energy channels, treated in acupuncture, and this heals and rejuvenates the whole body, creating physical, emotional, and mental harmony.

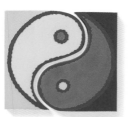

Dynamic balance

"Tai chi" is the name of the familiar yin-yang diagram which shows opposing forces in a state of dynamic balance. As an abbreviation of "tai chi chuan," the first part refers to the yin-yang balance, while "chuan" means "fist" and symbolizes martial art. So "tai chi chuan" means martial art based on the principles of yin and yang, the principles of harmonious balance.

No special equipment or uniform is needed and everyone, young and old, can gain peace of mind and strength of body from Tai Chi training and enjoy its healing benefits. After practicing it regularly people say they feel more balanced not only physically but mentally and emotionally, because Tai Chi is also a type of moving meditation. The development of Tai Chi is linked to Chinese philosophy, and after many years of regular practice it is possible to enter into a more spiritual state of being, but one does not have to be a Buddhist or a Daoist (Taoist) or to have any particular belief system or religion to benefit from it.

The central part of Tai Chi, and the main sequence to learn, is called the Form, and is a prearranged sequence of stylized self-defense movements, which are performed in a continuous flowing way. These relaxed movements release stress and invigorate the circulation of blood and qi (chi) energy, creating a sense of well-being.

WILL IT HELP?

• Tai Chi gently invigorates the circulation without straining the heart, making it beneficial for people with circulatory disorders.
• The gentle rotating of all the joints in the body helps maintain their flexibility, so Tai Chi is often recommended for those with arthritic and rheumatic conditions.
• Tai Chi practice increases the body's energy levels, without involving any strain, so it is suitable for older people and for those recovering from illness.
• Breathing is coordinated with every Tai Chi movement, so those practicing it find that their lungs get stronger and respiratory conditions are healed.

According to Chinese medicine, invisible energy channels called meridians run through the body, carrying qi (chi), or life force energy. For perfect physical and mental health, qi must be able to flow freely. There are 12 main meridians, which relate to different organs in the body: Lung, Spleen, Heart, Kidney, Pericardium, Liver, Large Intestine, Small Intestine, Stomach, Bladder, San Jiao, and Gallbladder.

 BENEFITS

• Tai Chi improves balance and coordination, strengthens circulation and respiration, and is a relaxing form of moving meditation.
• Tai Chi heals the mind, emotions, body, and spirit.
• It can be practiced indoors and out and can be easily incorporated into the day's routine.

 CAUTION

• The form of Tai Chi practiced simply for health is slow and easy to perform, and is safe for everybody. The form practiced for self-defense is very vigorous and is not suitable for anyone old or weak.

A complete Tai Chi routine may involve around fifty movements, and the sequence begins and ends with the body in the same position.

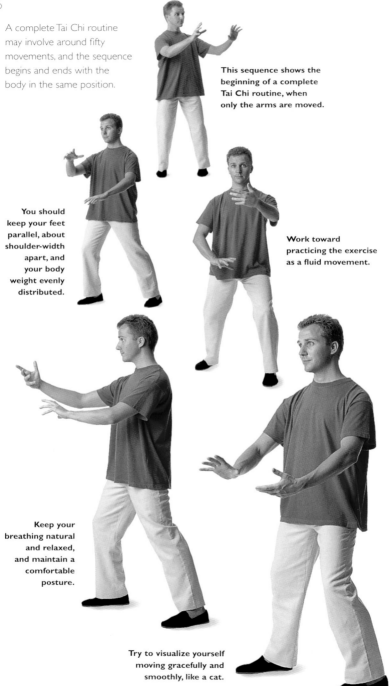

This sequence shows the beginning of a complete Tai Chi routine, when only the arms are moved.

You should keep your feet parallel, about shoulder-width apart, and your body weight evenly distributed.

Work toward practicing the exercise as a fluid movement.

Keep your breathing natural and relaxed, and maintain a comfortable posture.

Try to visualize yourself moving gracefully and smoothly, like a cat.

Yang Lu Chan

The most popular style of Tai Chi today is the Yang style, the version created by Yang Lu Chan (1799–1872). Yang Lu Chan was a short man of slight build, but through single-minded determination and continuous dedicated training he became an unequaled martial fighter with incredible spiritual force. He was taught Tai Chi by a descendant of Chang San Feng, and he expanded the system to include several new exercises which are now well-known.

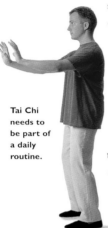

Tai Chi needs to be part of a daily routine.

Most people learn Tai Chi by attending a training class once or twice a week and practicing every day by themselves. Training every day is important because regular repetition of the movements keeps the body's qi (chi) energy flowing. If this energy flow is allowed to stagnate or become blocked then illness will develop.

Tai Chi in practice

Tai Chi consists of a series of movement sequences. As healing exercises, each movement strengthens and tones a different group of muscles, tendons, and joints. The rhythmic breathing also enhances blood circulation in the abdomen, speeding up the action of the intestines.

A complete Tai Chi routine takes about ten minutes, and progresses from movements involving only the arms and hands to movement of all the limbs in a graceful dancelike routine. It is possible to perform a free-style form of exercise based on Tai Chi that you invent as you go along, focusing on relaxed breathing and movement. This is simple to learn and will provide some of the benefits of a complete Tai Chi sequence.

 Is Tai Chi compatible with conventional medicine?
Tai Chi invigorates the body's natural energy and enhances general well-being, thus reducing the need for minor medical treatments.

 Is a practitioner necessary?
Initially you will need a teacher to show you the moves.

Chi Kung

Chi Kung, or Qi Gong, is an Ancient Chinese form of energy exercise, still widely practiced in modern China to prevent and heal disease and create balance in the body, mind, emotions, and spirit. In this self-healing system prescribed therapeutic postures are practiced every day.

Although about 2,000 different styles exist in mainland China, we can organize Chi Kung into five main types: holding-still postures, moving postures, breathing exercises, meditative practices, and leading the chi energy through the body with the mind. There are many reasons for practicing Chi Kung; as well as improving health and reducing stress it can be practiced as a form of meditation and as an aid to self-development or spiritual development.

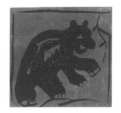

The Bear is one of the Five Animal Forms.

The history of Chi Kung

The practice of Chi Kung is thought to be at least 3,000 years old. It is illustrated in bronze tablets known as the Jin Wen from the Zhou dynasty (1100–221 BCE). It also appears in finds from Mawangdui in Changsha, the capital of Hunan Province, which include pieces of silk from the Western Han dynasty (206 BCE–CE 24) with painted figures of men and women practicing recognizable Chi Kung exercises. The style they are using is still practised today and is called the Five Animal Forms, with movements known as the Bear, the Ape, the Tiger, the Deer, and the Bird. Instructions on how to combine breathing with these movements were written on the silk.

In the Tang Dynasty (CE 618–907) Chi Kung exercises were widely used in medical treatments. Patients practiced prescribed exercises to help heal themselves and the physician used Chi Kung to transmit his healing energy to the patient. Today Chi Kung is becoming popular in the Western world, with many books, videos, and teachers available. Its benefits can be felt within a few weeks of practice if you train every day.

The Ape movement imitates the animal's quick, darting steps.

 WILL IT HELP?

• There are Chi Kung exercises for almost every known condition: respiratory, circulatory, digestive, glandular, and sexual problems can all be healed.

• Through Chi Kung the immune system can be strengthened and the rate of recovery from illness increased.

• Over time daily training can lead to a feeling of well-being, emotional calm, and clarity of mind.

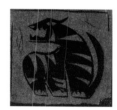

The Tiger Form involves making clawlike shapes with the hands.

 BENEFITS

• General improvement in health, more energy, and greater peace of mind.

• Healing of specific illnesses is possible if an appropriate Chi Kung system is used.

 CAUTION

• Although Chi Kung exercises can be learned from books and from videos, it is always best to begin with lessons from an advanced practitioner.

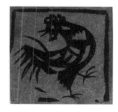

For the Bird movement, the arms are spread out like wings.

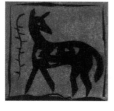

The Deer movement strengthens the legs.

CHI KUNG POSTURE   An example of a Chi Kung still standing posture is shown below. When practicing these postures it is important to pay attention to your body structure. The feet should be shoulder width apart and parallel to each other. The knees are slightly bent, and pushed out so as to make the shins vertical. Your body weight should be focused at the point where you tie your shoelaces, where the shin bone meets the top of the foot. Gently curl your toes under.

Make sure your spine is straight and vertical, and roll your tailbone under, which has the effect of making the lumbar region of your spine straight. Tuck your chin in slightly to help straighten the top of your spine. (Imagine that there is a thread attached to the crown of your head pulling you up.) The shoulders and belly should be relaxed and the arms should maintain a circular shape, as if you were hugging a large tree. Put the tongue on the roof of the mouth at the front, as when pronouncing the letter "L."

MENTAL STATE   Chi Kung helps the mind to attain a peaceful and harmonious state. As the chi (qi) energy flows without restriction you find that you feel relaxed and calm deep down inside. The person learning Chi Kung is taught to keep a little attention always focused on an area called the "tan tien," just below and behind the navel. This is a major energy center in the body where, in the theory supporting Chi Kung, we can accumulate and store our chi (qi) energy.

Chi Kung postures help you to focus on your body shape and breathing pattern so as to control the flow of chi.

Is Chi Kung compatible with conventional medicine?
Chi Kung invigorates the body's natural energy and enhances general well-being, thus reducing the need for minor medical treatments. It can also address specific conditions in concert with conventional treatment.

Is a practitioner necessary?
You will need a teacher initially to show you the exercises.

NATURAL THERAPIES

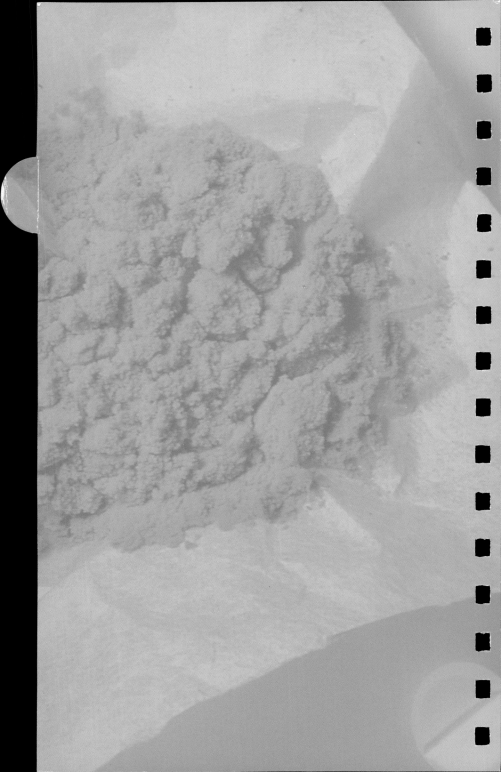

Probably the first thing that springs to mind when complementary therapies are mentioned are the therapies based on natural remedies. Herbalism has a long and honorable history; indeed, for thousands of years, herbs were the only medicine available, so it is unsurprising that there exists a huge body of knowledge and expertise about their properties and applications. Although eclipsed by the wonder-drug culture of the 20th century, herbalism is gradually reestablishing its status as a useful therapeutic tool. Homeopathy is a much younger therapy, dating from the mid-18th century. Although homeopathy is based on remedies made from natural sources, its underlying philosophy is more abstract than that of herbalism. Both therapies are generally safe for home treatment, but if you suffer from a specific medical condition you should seek expert guidance from a qualified practitioner.

Homeopathy

Homeopathy is a holistic system of medicine devised by a German physician, Samuel Hahnemann (1755–1843). Homeopaths take into account their patients' physical, emotional, and mental characteristics, as well as full details of their symptoms when ill, including seemingly unrelated ones. The treatment is by infinitesimally tiny dilutions of a variety of substances prepared (usually) in tablet form. Many are substances that would be harmful or toxic if taken in any other form, but the method of producing them—known as potentization—renders them into a harmless but effective medicine, which has no undesirable side effects. The operative principle is that a substance that could cause the symptoms of an illness in a healthy person can cure the same symptoms when given in a homeopathically potentized form to a sick person. The treatment works by stimulating the body to cure itself.

The basics of the homeopath's treatment kit have not really changed since homeopathy was invented.

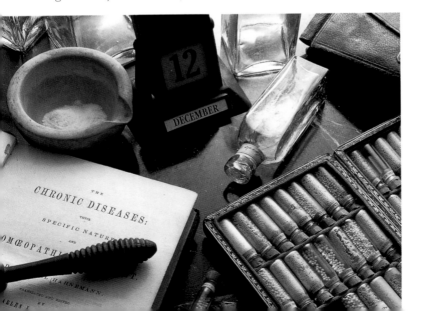

WILL IT HELP?

Homeopathy is suitable for chronic, long-term conditions, sudden, acute problems, and a number of emergency situations. It can be used to treat:

CHRONIC
- headaches, migraines
- allergies, rashes, and skin conditions
- recurrent digestive problems
- arthritis, rheumatism
- asthma and other respiratory problems
- menopausal difficulties
- PMT and menstrual problems

ACUTE
- coughs, colds
- childhood infections
- stomach problems
- teething

FIRST AID
- insect stings and bites
- minor burns and scalds
- motion sickness
- shock that accompanies accidents and mishaps

 BENEFITS

- The dilution of homeopathic remedies means that there are no side effects.
- The treatment is completely safe and can never lead to further illness.
- The remedies are tasteless and easy to take and can be taken in tablet or liquid form.

CAUTION

- Coffee, peppermint, camphor, menthol, eucalyptus, and other strong-smelling substances act against the remedy and should not be used when taking homeopathic remedies or for four weeks afterward. You should not smoke while having homeopathic treatment.

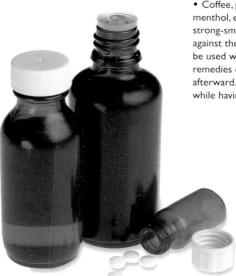

Homeopathic remedies are given as tablets or in liquid form.

How homeopathy developed

In 1796 Samuel Hahnemann was translating a medical book on a medicine derived from Peruvian bark, or cinchona (*Cinchona officinalis*) that was used to treat malaria. He was struck by the fact that this plant extract cured symptoms similar to those it would cause in someone who did not have malaria. Hahnemann then decided to experiment by taking some cinchona himself and subsequently developed symptoms of malaria. He found that when he took a diluted dose of cinchona all these symptoms cleared. From this early research he went on to devise numerous experiments, that he performed on himself and a number of volunteers, all of which confirmed the principle that a substance that causes disease symptoms can be used to treat the same symptoms successfully if administered in a suitably diluted and potentized form. This principle Hahnemann called the Law of Similars.

It came to light during the course of these experiments that individuals react differently to treatment according to their types, and part of the homeopathic physician's skill is to match remedy exactly to patient as well as to disease. The main principle is to treat each patient as an individual because no two patients are alike. They are each made up of particular characteristics, which can be tabulated to some extent—their height, weight, eye color, and even their reactions and dispositions—so it follows that individuals will react to medicines differently. From this, homeopathy developed into a system of medicine by which the remedies are prescribed strictly according to the individual requirements of each patient.

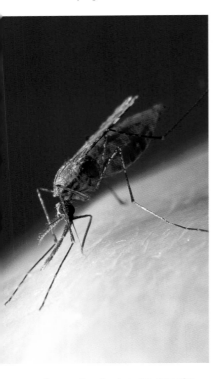

As a carrier of malaria, the mosquito continues to threaten human health. Hahnemann's homeopathic investigations were triggered by his own observations of malaria treatment.

Consulting a homeopath

To achieve this remedy–patient match a homeopathic practitioner will take a very detailed history, asking not only about the patient's health but also about the health of parents, grandparents, brothers, and sisters. He or she will also want to know about the patient's temperament, likes and

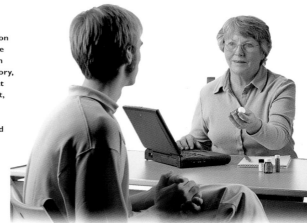

As with most complementary therapies consultation time is generous. The practitioner takes an exhaustive case history, asking questions that can, to a new patient, seem irrelevant. Practitioners also explain diagnosis and the remedies prescribed.

dislikes, lifestyle, exercise habits, and diet, which can have a great bearing on the patient's health. The practitioner may carry out tests such as testing the urine and taking the blood pressure, and some homeopaths use complementary diagnostic aids such as iridology. When the homeopath has taken the patient's history then he or she will use a given procedure to arrive at the remedy most suitable to that individual.

To find the most suitable remedy the practitioner "repertorizes" the case, using a book called a repertory, which lists virtually every symptom known, together with a list of the most suitable remedies for each. A chart is made up (see pages 56–7), using each symptom, to give a complete overall picture of the case, and it becomes apparent which remedies should be most useful for the patient. Many homeopaths today use a computer to carry out the repertorizing. The use of a chart makes it possible for patients to repertorize their own cases and this can be practiced without a practitioner for nonserious conditions. However, if the condition is chronic or of a more serious nature then the help of a practitioner must always be sought.

Remedy sources

Hahnemann's remedies came from the animal, vegetable, and mineral kingdoms. Today many more new ingredients for remedies are being discovered; some are also made from synthetic chemical compounds, and some, called nosodes, from the bacteria or virus that actually cause disease. For example, the tuberculinum remedy is made from the bacillus that causes tuberculosis. Since remedies are diluted hundreds of times there is no danger in them.

CHILDREN'S CONDITIONS

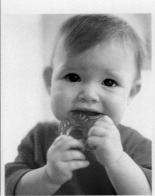

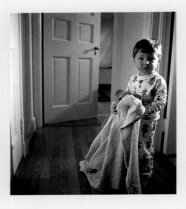

Teething
Chamomilla: when the child is irritable and wants to be held; one cheek pale and one cheek flushed; loose bowel motions
Aconite: if the child is feverish and in great pain
Belladonna: when the child is irritable, with high temperature; flushed cheeks

Bed-wetting
Sabadilla: for general bladder weakness
Sulfur: for children who sweat a lot at night, are irritable, untidy
Gelsemium: useful in nervous, hysterical children
Lycopodium: more useful for boys

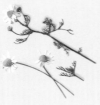

CHAMOMILE

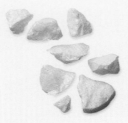

SULFUR

Home treatment for children

Homeopathic remedies are perfectly safe for treating children at home. Remember that symptoms may become worse before they get better;. However, if you are at all concerned about your child's health, contact a doctor. If a child has any of the following, get medical help immediately, because meningitis may be indicated: severe headache, vomiting, stiff neck, sensitivity to light, lethargy, or a rash that does not disappear when pressed with a glass.

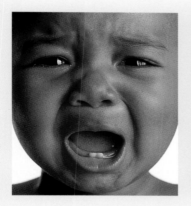

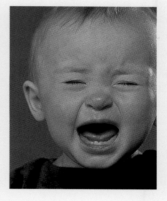

Sickness and diarrhea

Arsenicum: for severe diarrhea nearly always accompanied by sickness
Pulsatilla: when bowel motions are changeable, worse evenings, and child is weepy
China: for pale, mucous diarrhea, often worse after eating fruit

Earache

Belladonna: for a throbbing earache, with high temperature, redness, no thirst
Aconite: for an earache with acute onset, pain, and fever, eased by heat applied locally

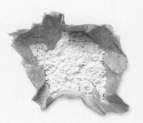

ARSENIOUS OXIDE

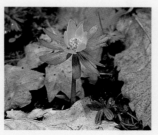

ACONITE

Preparing remedies

Homeopathic remedies are made from substances that have been found by clinical experience to stimulate a curative action. They are prepared stage by stage and not all at once. The dilution of the substances to infinitesimally small proportions during their preparation is one of the unique features of homeopathy and is a safeguard against toxicity and side effects. At the same time this dilution of the remedies adds to their power to stimulate a response. This is thought to be because as each successive dilution, or potency, is strongly agitated by vigorous, rhythmic shaking (succussion) it is given a vitality that aids the patient's recovery. For this reason the succussion process is known as "vitalizing" or "potentizing."

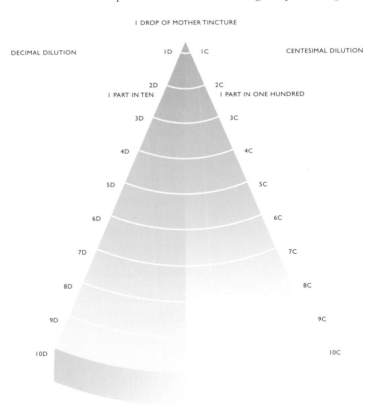

I DROP OF MOTHER TINCTURE

DECIMAL DILUTION   ID   IC   CENTESIMAL DILUTION

2D   2C
I PART IN TEN   I PART IN ONE HUNDRED

3D   3C

4D   4C

5D   5C

6D   6C

7D   7C

8D   8C

9D   9C

10D   10C

Two scales of dilution are used in preparing homeopathic remedies. The decimal scale is used for multiple remedies and the centesimal scale for single remedies.

Scales of dilution

There are two scales of dilution used in preparation: the decimal scale and the centesimal scale. Dilutions on the decimal scale are made by taking one drop of a mother tincture (the first dilution of the original substance) and mixing it with ten drops of pure alcohol substance. This solution is called 1d (d standing for decimal). The solution is left to infuse and is shaken at intervals. One drop of this is then removed and the operation repeated with it (this is called 2d) and so on. This scale of dilution is normally used in what is known as complex homeopathy, where more than one remedy is put in the prescription.

The other scale used, centesimal, follows the same procedure but one drop is used per 100 drops of mother tincture (to give the dilution known as 1c) and then the process is repeated as before. Homeopathic practitioners may use up to 1M or 10M or even higher (1M is 1000 x dilution and 10M is 10,000 x). This is the system normally used in classical homeopathy, where only one remedy is used.

Over the past few years another method, that of descending potencies, has been demonstrated by Pritam Singh Ghattaoraya, who closely studied the original work of Hahnemann. Many homeopaths now use this method of descending potencies, either changing the potency each day or, in some cases, giving remedies in different potency each hour or at intervals during the day, sometimes together with changing the remedies as well. This method can be used with great success but it should only be on the prescription of a homeopathic practitioner.

 Is homeopathy compatible with conventional medicine?
Homeopathic remedies contain almost no trace of the original substance from which they were made, and act on an energy level rather than a biochemical level. They are therefore perfectly safe to use in conjunction with conventional medications.

 Is a practitioner necessary?
For serious conditions, particularly if there are children involved, it is always a good idea to get expert advice from a qualified homeopath who will be able to identify the best remedy for the situation. However, home treatment is perfectly safe when the patient has sufficient knowledge of their own condition.

Herbal medicine

Herbal medicine is arguably the oldest system of medicine on the planet, and it is viewed on a global scale, still the most commonly used type of medicine. Over millennia each culture on earth has developed its own knowledge of indigenous healing plants and their characteristics and uses. Herbs still offer a wide range of self-treatment options for minor day-to-day dis-orders and can also be used to tackle more serious conditions. In the West today we are seeing a resurgence in the professional prac-tice of herbal medicine, founded on growing public interest in treatment that is supportive and natural, and that causes few side effects.

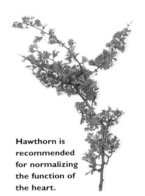

Hawthorn is recommended for normalizing the function of the heart.

Conventional medicine evolved substantially out of the herbal tradition and many of today's drugs—such as aspirin (from willow and meadowsweet), morphine (from the opium poppy), and even the contraceptive pill (from wild yam)—were originally derived from plants. The crucial difference between herbal medicine and a drug derived from a plant is that the for-mer uses the whole plant (or plant part) from which it is produced, mini-mally processed, while the latter is made by extracting one small, therapeutically active ingredient from the plant, discarding the rest.

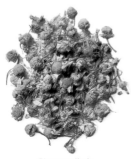

Chamomile is a sedative.

Medical herbalists contend that the matter dis-carded in the preparation of modern drugs is not extraneous. Instead, it represents many cofactors which work alongside the main active principle in the plant to make the herbal remedy safer, and more gently effective. The wealth of traditional experience on which herbalism is founded is now being supplemented by high-quality research, serving to raise the profile of herbal medicine and bring it right back as a major part of mainstream healthcare.

WILL IT HELP?

- Herbs characteristically have a positive effect on general bodily functioning and promote a sense of well-being, traditionally known as a "tonic" effect.
- Herbal medicine can help the majority of problems you might consult your doctor about and can be used by people of all ages.
- Its wide scope includes the treatment of infections, allergies, asthma, high blood pressure, arthritis, migraines, insomnia, eczema, digestive disorders, and gynecological problems.
- It is becoming increasingly valued for its role in treating stress, depression, chronic fatigue, and impaired immunity.

 BENEFITS

- Plant medicines are gentle and well tolerated. They support natural body processes, working with the body's own defense system.
- They are nonaddictive and do not promote dependency, making them easy to withdraw from.
- The benefits gathered from a course of treatment are profound and long-lasting. Improvements persist after the medicine has stopped.

 CAUTION

- Herbs are powerful healing agents. A very small minority of them are potentially toxic and should be taken only on expert advice.
- It is not advisable to gather your own wild herbs because of the danger of misidentifying species and the risks of contamination by herbicides or pollution, and because of adverse impact on the environment.
- Vulnerable groups of people, such as small children, the elderly, and pregnant or breastfeeding women, should always seek professional advice before taking herbs.

Lavender has many applications.

Herbal traditions

Owing to its great age and widespread use, various approaches to the practice of herbal medicine have evolved. Some traditions, such as Chinese herbal medicine and Indian Ayurveda, persist virtually intact to this day. Others, notably the Western tradition, have been fragmented by cultural and political developments. All, however, share a basic unifying principle, in that they each place central value on stimulating the body's innate self-healing power, known as "chi" (Chinese), "prana" (Indian), or the "vital force" (Western). A core feature of the philosophy of herbalism is the emphasis on helping the body to recover balance, adding strength to its natural healing processes. The herbalist acknowledges the body's capacity for health and seeks to support and assist it, not to dominate or override it.

Garlic is a powerful natural antiseptic, antibiotic, fungicide, and expectorant.

Herbalism respects the complexity of the human organism and the variation among individuals. Similarly, plants are tremendously complex in their makeup and consequently they interact therapeutically with us in a very harmonious way. The herbalist's approach to the patient is both holistic (taking account of the person as a whole, looking at the current problem, and the person's medical history in great detail), and naturopathic (deciding how best to rally the innate self-healing powers). The herbalist uses the whole plant to treat the whole person.

THE RANGE OF HERBAL POWERS The medicinal action of herbs extends across a wide spectrum. At one end are those that are essentially foods with therapeutic effect. These include garlic and onions, which can lower cholesterol and are antiseptic; beets, which stimulates the immune system; and culinary herbs such as thyme, sage, and basil, which possess antibiotic and antiphlegm properties. Next comes a very large selection of herbs that have no real food use but which are safe, gentle, and medicinally active, such as elecampane for chest infection and hawthorn for the heart and circulation. A small group at the opposite end of the spectrum are very active, strong herbs that are potentially harmful, but which can be of great use when prescribed by a qualified medical herbalist. This includes yellow jasmine, which can be used to treat pain.

PREPARING HERBS FOR USE The modern medical herbalist uses traditional plant preparations of roots, leaves, flowers, fruits, or seeds. These preparations retain the majority of the plant's constituents, and so work in a balanced and safe way. Usually a number of herbs are combined in one prescription to act synergistically. This means that the combined effect of the total medicine is more than the simple sum of its separate herbal parts. The main ways in which herbs are prepared are described on pages 66–7.

Self-help

It is always advisable to consult a qualified medical herbalist for problems that are serious or recurring, but it is also possible to use herbal medicine very successfully as a self-help treatment. With a little research and some common sense a variety of common ailments can be treated. Many minor health problems occur during the course of our lives and it is helpful to have a little knowledge of herbal medicine and a stock of remedies to hand to tackle these conditions as they arise, for both our families and ourselves.

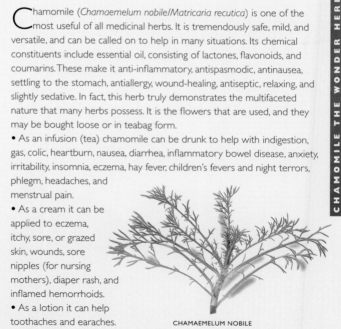

Chamomile (*Chamaemelum nobile/Matricaria recutica*) is one of the most useful of all medicinal herbs. It is tremendously safe, mild, and versatile, and can be called on to help in many situations. Its chemical constituents include essential oil, consisting of lactones, flavonoids, and coumarins. These make it anti-inflammatory, antispasmodic, antinausea, settling to the stomach, antiallergy, wound-healing, antiseptic, relaxing, and slightly sedative. In fact, this herb truly demonstrates the multifaceted nature that many herbs possess. It is the flowers that are used, and they may be bought loose or in teabag form.

• As an infusion (tea) chamomile can be drunk to help with indigestion, gas, colic, heartburn, nausea, diarrhea, inflammatory bowel disease, anxiety, irritability, insomnia, eczema, hay fever, children's fevers and night terrors, phlegm, headaches, and menstrual pain.

• As a cream it can be applied to eczema, itchy, sore, or grazed skin, wounds, sore nipples (for nursing mothers), diaper rash, and inflamed hemorrhoids.

• As a lotion it can help toothaches and earaches.

CHAMAEMELUM NOBILE

CHAMOMILE THE WONDER HERB

The most famous of all physicians, the Ancient Greek Hippocrates, said: "Let food be your medicine and medicine be your food." And the best way to start with healing plants is to appreciate their importance in the diet. Incorporating medicinal foods is an effective way of helping to prevent illness in the first place. Culinary herbs and spices are both health-promoting and tasty. For example, cayenne pepper and ginger are warming to the circulation, cinnamon calms the digestion, and turmeric is anti-inflammatory. Fruits such as black grapes and blackberries, and vegetables such as carrots and red peppers have antioxidant properties, which protect against cell damage and may also help to prevent some forms of cancer.

TREATING COMMON AILMENTS From using herbs in food preparation one can progress to building up a knowledge of useful herbs one by one. Consider the recurrent problems you tend to suffer from and the conditions your children are likely to encounter, and then explore the herbs that are relevant for your own likely needs. Some examples of herbal preparations that are useful for the home are:

• marshmallow syrup to soothe dry coughs
• thyme and licorice syrup for wet, phlegmy coughs
• infusion (tea) made with equal parts elderflower, yarrow, and peppermint for colds
• calendula cream or ointment for cuts, bruises, insect bites, and burns
• infusion (tea) made from fennel or lemon balm for indigestion
• limeflower infusion (tea) for insomnia, muscular tension, headaches, and anxiety

SOME USEFUL HERBS	Common name	Botanical name	Action	Uses
	Echinacea	*Echinacea purpurea*	Stimulates the immune system	Colds, influenza, skin infections
	Siberian ginseng	*Eleutherococcus senticosus*	Improves stamina	Fatigue, tiredness
	Agrimony	*Agrimonia eupatoria*	Astringent	Diarrhea, loose bowel motions
	Cleavers	*Galium aparine*	Cleansing	Eczema, itchy skin
	Eyebright	*Euphrasia officinalis*	Soothes mucous membranes	Hay fever, conjunctivitis

Consulting a practitioner

Although you can treat minor, everyday health problems at home, you should consult a qualified medical herbalist, or a doctor, for all significant health problems and for any minor problems that are failing to clear up. Consultation is also advised for babies and young children, elderly people, and women who are pregnant or breastfeeding. You should also seek the advice of a medical herbalist before treating yourself if you are taking conventional medication. Many herbs have potent pharmacological activity which may potentiate (increase the action of) conventional medicines or react negatively with them.

A typical first consultation will last about an hour and include the taking of a very detailed case history, together with any relevant physical examinations. As well as herbal medicine you may be given advice on diet and lifestyle. Follow-up visits will usually be needed every two to four weeks after the initial visit, and generally take about half an hour. Typically, treatment for acute, short-lived problems takes from one to six weeks while treatment for chronic, long-term conditions takes from three months to a year.

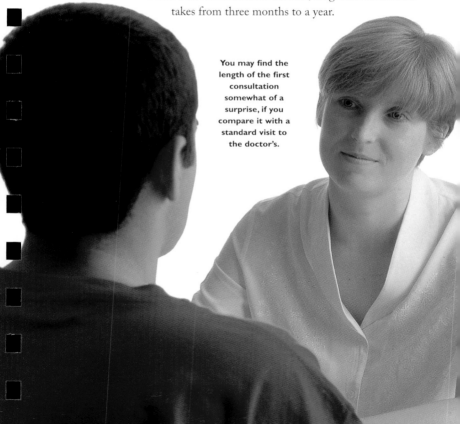

You may find the length of the first consultation somewhat of a surprise, if you compare it with a standard visit to the doctor's.

Using herbs at home

Many types of herbal preparation are available, including tablets, capsules, tinctures (liquid extracts in a water/alcohol solution), syrups, juices, creams, and poultices. For self-help it is usually best to use dried herbs made into an infusion (tea). This enables you to make effective treatments and actually see what the herb looks like and get to know its taste and smell.

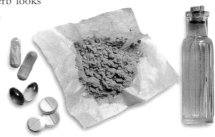

BUYING HERBS Buy herbs from a reputable supplier who is likely to have a quick turnover. When selecting herbs ensure that they have a good natural color, that they appear crisp, clean, and dry, and that they smell fresh. Store them in dark glass jars with lids or in a

Herbal medicine takes various forms, some of which can be stored more successfully than others.

heavy, sealed brown paper bag, and label them clearly so that there will be no confusion about the contents. Make a note also of the date you bought them. Keep the herbs out of direct sunlight and away from damp and heat. They will keep for up to a year.

PREPARING HERBS There are two ways of preparing herbs ready to drink: by infusion and by decoction. Infusion, by steeping the herbs in hot water, is the usual way to make a tea. This is suitable for soft plant parts, such as thin leaves, flowers, and fine seeds, which readily release their constituents into water. The herbs should be allowed to steep with the container covered with a clean lid or saucer, to prevent the steam from escaping. Use the decoction method for hard plant parts, such as thick, waxy leaves, roots, fruits, and hard seeds, which do not easily give up their healing compounds into solution. The methods of preparation are illustrated in the steps opposite.

TAKING YOUR HERBAL TEA The standard dose for adults, using dried herbs (by infusion or decoction), is two teaspoons (2 x 5ml spoons) to one cup (about 150ml) of water. Normally one whole cup should be drunk three times a day. If it is inconvenient to make tea on three separate occasions during the day (perhaps because you are out at work) you can prepare all three cups at once in the morning, drink the first cup and pour the remainder into a thermos to use later.

MAKING AN INFUSION

1 Add two teaspoons (2 x 5ml spoons) of dried herbs per cup to the teapot (preferably kept specially for herbs). Glass teapots or cafetières are ideal since they allow you to watch the tea infusing.

2 Pour the measured amount of just-boiled water onto the herbs, cover, and leave the infusion to brew for ten minutes.

3 Pour the infusion through a tea strainer and drink it while it is still hot. Try to savor the taste and the aroma as you drink.

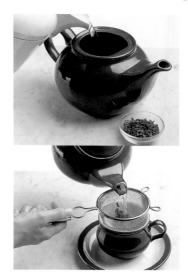

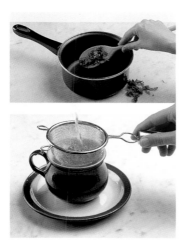

MAKING A DECOCTION

1 Add two teaspoons (2 x 5ml spoons) of the herbal ingredients to a pan. Use a lidded pan made of glass, enamel, or stainless steel.

2 Pour on the measured amount of cold water and bring slowly to the boil. Simmer for 15 minutes with the lid on to prevent evaporation.

3 Pour the decoction through a tea strainer and drink while still hot. Find a quiet moment to relax and fully enjoy your herbal tea.

 Is herbal medicine compatible with conventional medicine?
Medical herbalism can be compatible with conventional medicine. Herbs can be used either as an alternative to orthodox drugs or alongside them as complementary treatment.

 Is a practitioner necessary?
A practitioner is recommended but not always essential.

Flower remedies

Flower remedies were first developed by a homeopathic physician, Dr. Edward Bach, in the 1920s. Recognizing that negative mental states had an adverse effect on people's health, he used his experience of homeopathy to identify flowers that could be used to address particular states of mind. Although they have no identifiable biochemical action, flower remedies draw on the essential vibrational life force of the flowers used to make them to harmonize mind, body, and spirit.

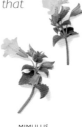

MIMULUS

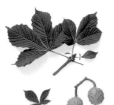

Horse Chestnut is a remedy for anxiety.

Using flower remedies

The 38 Bach Flower Remedies are the best-known collection of remedies. Each addresses a particular emotional state. Cherry Plum, for example, addresses irrational thoughts or behavior, Gentian is for despondency, and Willow helps with feelings of self-pity and resentment. All the remedies are intended to restore emotional balance and encourage well-being.

Flower remedies are sold in stock bottles, in which the essence of the flower is preserved in brandy. It is possible to use a single remedy, but it is often better to create a personal remedy using a combination of essences, mixing two drops of each together in 1 fl oz (30ml) of water. Flower remedies are not addictive or dangerous, and can be used by children, the elderly, and pregnant women.

 Are flower remedies compatible with conventional medicine?
Flower remedies address the emotional imbalances underlying illness, and can augment conventional treatments.

 Is a practitioner necessary?
Flower remedies were created for people to use themselves, but some homeopaths and herbalists also use them.

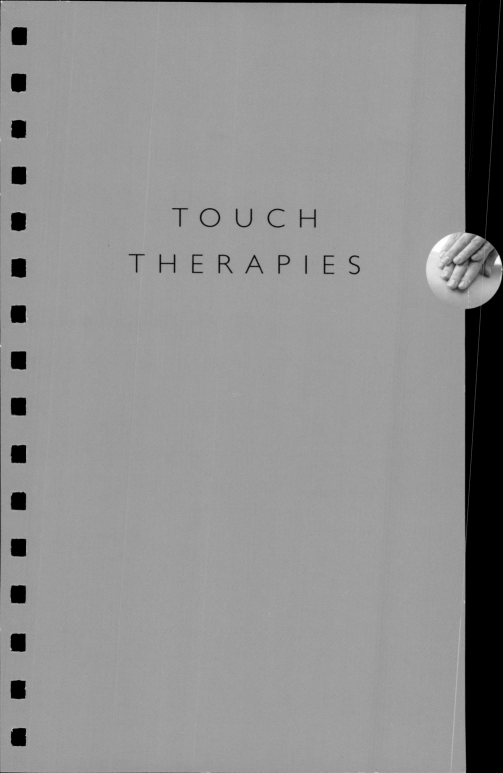

TOUCH
THERAPIES

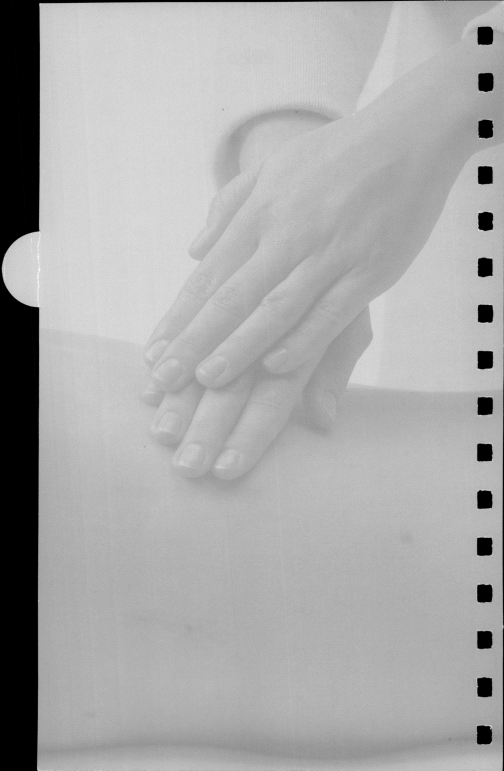

Rubbing it better is the oldest healing technique of all, one that is practiced almost unconsciously by all of us at some time in our lives. Massage, aromatherapy, reflexology, and Shiatsu are based on the therapeutic touch; all are ancient therapies, based on tried and tested methods, and enjoy a great deal of success in reviving tense muscles and tired minds. Massage, the most mainstream of these therapies, is well known for its effect on strains and injuries; aromatherapy adds mood-changing scent to massage; reflexology, now extremely popular, concentrates on the soles of the feet and the palms of the hands as gateways to the rest of the body; and Shiatsu, a Japanese massage therapy, shares some principles with Chinese acupressure. A practitioner is essential for the full benefit of all four therapies, although it is possible to self-administer a limited amount of massage, aromatherapy, and reflexology.

Massage

Massage is derived from the most basic form of touch therapy. The English word comes from the French for "to rub"—a natural human reflex when there is pain or injury. This natural tendency to rub something better has been formalized over thousands of years to develop into the system of therapeutic touch that we know as massage today. In the West, the type that is most familiar to us is Swedish massage, founded by Per Henrick Ling in the early 19th century. This form of massage had became popular throughout Europe by the end of that century and is now an established part of health and beauty therapy.

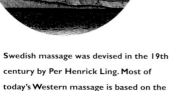

Swedish massage was devised in the 19th century by Per Henrick Ling. Most of today's Western massage is based on the work of this Scandinavian practitioner.

The history of massage

The Ancient Greek physician Hippocrates is said to have recommended a daily scented bath and a massage as a key to health and well-being. The practice of massage (anointing the skin with oil) is mentioned in texts as old as the Bible and the Koran, but it is thought that massage was performed in China as early as 3000 BCE. Massage techniques were used by early Eastern and Middle Eastern cultures as part of daily health programs and massage is still commonly used in those parts of the world today.

WILL IT HELP?

• A massage can help a wide range of both physical and psychological conditions, wherever there is muscular tension in the body.
• Common aches and pains can be soothed by a massage, including neck and shoulder tension and backaches.
• The relaxing effect of a massage helps to improve the flow of lymph, enhancing the functioning of the body's immune system.
• It can help improve circulation, and relieve conditions attributed to poor circulation.
• Stress, anxiety, insomnia, headaches, and migraines can all be alleviated.
• Digestive problems such as constipation and gas can be relieved with an abdominal massage.
• Menstrual pain can be eased and soothed.

 BENEFITS

• Relaxes muscular tension, eases stress, and promotes relaxation and sleep.
• Gives comfort, support, and reassurance through touch.
• May reduce the need for medication for stress and pain relief.
• Can also be used to promote intimacy between couples.

 CAUTION

• For a therapeutic massage find a qualified practitioner, who will have been trained in physiology and who will check that there are no contraindications to treatment.
• Do not have a massage when you have a high temperature.
• Do not have a massage over broken skin, broken bones, bruises, or unexplained lumps and bumps.
• Check for allergies: do not use a nut-based oil for a massage if in doubt.
• Approach an abdominal massage during pregnancy with great caution. Essential oils should not be used in pregnancy (see Aromatherapy, page 83).
• If you are being treated for a medical condition do not undergo a massage without a doctor's advice.

What is a massage?

A massage can be vigorous or gentle, stimulating or sedating, and is usually performed using just the hands. To enable them to move smoothly over the skin and work on the muscles, tendons, and ligaments, a carrier oil, cream, lotion, or talcum powder, is used. Massage may be used on the whole or part of the body, according to its therapeutic aims. The person being massaged usually lies on a firm treatment couch, although anyone who is ill or unable to lie flat may be worked on in bed or in a chair.

This natural therapy should be an enjoyable and relaxing experience. However, some people do not like being touched except by someone with whom they are intimate, and people from different cultures have different views on touch and massage and these feelings need to be respected. A qualified practitioner will be aware of any likely reserve, and will work tactfully to build up trust.

DIFFERENT FORMS OF MASSAGE   There are two main varieties of massage, apart from Swedish massage:

• Deep tissue massage is good for long-standing deep muscular problems. It works in a more penetrating way than Swedish massage.

• Sports massage works on specific areas of the body where there have been injuries.

These two types of treatment are generally too strong to be used all over the body at one time and are focused to assist the injured area.

Massage movements

Massage involves a variety of movements, some designed to stimulate and some to relax. During a general body massage these are usually performed in a set order, starting with long, slow, relaxing strokes. The main techniques are stroking, circling, kneading, hacking, cupping, and feathering.

STROKING   This is performed with the fingers held together and the thumbs open, over the entire surface of the area being massaged, with the hand molded to the shape of the body. The strokes are long and flowing and the pressure may vary from light to deep.

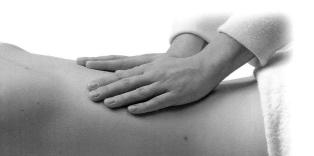

A massage begins
with long, slow,
relaxing strokes.

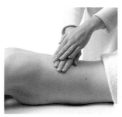

Fingertip circling using the even pressure of both hands.

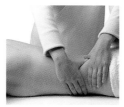

Kneading works on the superficial muscle.

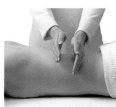

Hacking relieves muscular tension.

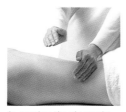

In cupping, the air caught under the hand provides a gentle pressure.

The massage is finished off with the finger-tip technique of feathering.

CIRCLING Finger and thumb circles are performed with the tips of the fingers or thumbs making small, slow, and rhythmical circles. Palm circles are performed with the palms of the hand making broad, slow, and rhythmical circles.

KNEADING This is an action similar to kneading bread dough. The whole hand picks up and kneads the superficial muscle. Rhythmical movements and alternating hands are used.

HACKING Using the sides of the hands, with wrists relaxed, a short, sharp movement is applied over the muscle to release tension.

CUPPING This uses cupped hands alternating on the muscle, making a sound like that of horse's hooves. It applies a gentle pressure to the area being treated as air is caught under the hand.

FEATHERING This consists of very light, stroking motions with the fingertips on the surface of the skin. No pressure is applied.

In a massage pressure and friction move the muscles and skin to release tension and treat ligaments and tendons. Moving the hands with pressure on the body helps the muscles to move freely, thus improving their elasticity and the flexibility of the body part and allowing any organs underneath to function better. For example, massaging the abdomen can ease constipation, while massaging the head, neck, and shoulders can relieve a headache.

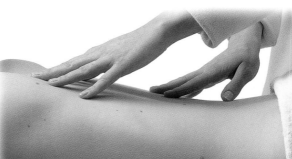

Massage at home

Tension and bad posture cause backaches and neck pain. It is possible to master the basic massage techniques and the order of using them so that you can give a simple massage to a friend or partner at home, to help to soothe away stiffness and pain, or simply as an aid to relaxation.

Before you start make sure that the room is warm and draft-free and that your nails are short and smooth. Have at least two bath towels ready, one for the person to lie on and the other to cover the parts not being massaged. You will need a plain carrier oil such as sunflower or almond oil, according to preference, and a padded, firm surface for the person receiving the massage to lie on. (The floor will do, but then you will have to kneel. A bed is usually not supportive enough: if you do use a bed it must be a very firm one, and preferably a single one so that you can reach the person from both sides.)

In general, massage is done in a slow, relaxed, and rhythmical manner, in a continuous flow of movement, and keeping at least one hand on the person being massaged when moving from one part of the body to another, or from one type of massage touch to another. Ensure that the person receiving the massage is in a comfortable position, warm, and relaxed. Clothing should be removed from the area to be massaged.
Be aware of your own body when giving massage:
• Keep a straight back
• Let the movements come from your pelvis, not just your shoulders, as this makes it less tiring on the arms and more effective.

A simple back massage

Get two bath towels and place one underneath the person to be massaged. Position the person on his or her front with the head to one side and cover the parts of the body that are not going to be massaged with a towel. Stand (or kneel) at the person's head.

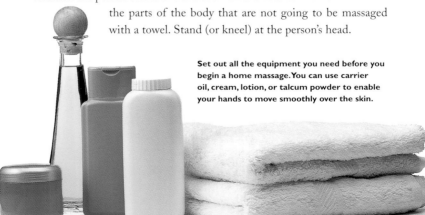

Set out all the equipment you need before you begin a home massage. You can use carrier oil, cream, lotion, or talcum powder to enable your hands to move smoothly over the skin.

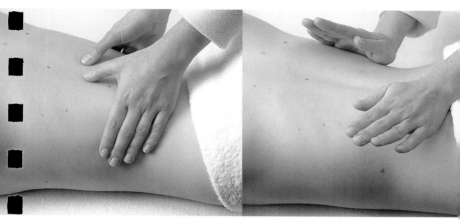

Relax the muscles of each vertebra using thumb circles.

Pressure is applied to the back in circular movements with the palms of the hands.

STROKING MOVEMENT I   Begin the massage by placing your hands either side of the spine at the top of the back, with fingers together and facing the buttocks, allowing the thumbs to cross. Run your hands down the back along each side of the spine, applying pressure with the whole of your hands except your thumbs. On the lower back, separate the hands and run them up toward the head along the side of the back. Repeat this movement three to five times, finishing at the top of the spine.

THUMB CIRCLES MOVEMENT 2   Place your thumbs either side of the spine, resting the other fingers on the back. Rotate your thumbs three times on the muscle beside each vertebra, as you gradually work your way down the back. When you have reached as far as you can, separate your hands and slide them up the sides of the back. Repeat three to five times.

PALM CIRCLES MOVEMENT 3   Rest the left-hand palm on the right upper back, and the right-hand palm on the left upper back. Leaving the left hand in place, rotate the right hand down the back in medium-sized circles. When at the bottom, slide the hand back up the right side and repeat three to five times. Repeat this movement on the other side.

STROKING MOVEMENT 4   Place your hands either side of the spine with the fingers together facing the buttocks, and allowing the thumbs to cross. Run your hands down the back beside the spine and along the lower back. Separate the hands and run up the side of the back. Repeat this movement three to five times, this time finishing at the base of the spine.

FINISH   Cover the person, and allow them to rest for five minutes.

Foot massage

This is an easy and effective massage to aid general relaxation. The feet
have numerous small bones and muscles, as well as nerve endings from all
the major nerves. They take the strain whenever we walk or stand, and
can retain a lot of tension. A foot massage can prevent or alleviate many
problems, keep the feet flexible, and soothe aches and pains.

The person to be treated should sit barefoot in a chair with their feet
up. Place a towel under their feet and fold it over so that both are covered.
Put some oil on your hands and rub together to warm it. Uncover one foot.

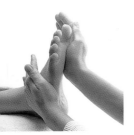
Movement 1
Stroking

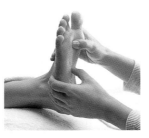
Movement 2
Thumb kneading

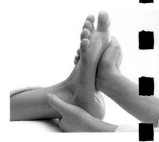
Movement 3
Palm kneading

STROKING MOVEMENT 1   Hold the foot between your two hands for
a few seconds as a kind of greeting. Using the flat of your hands, slowly
and rhythmically rub the upper surface of the foot with one hand and the
sole with the other. Repeat this 10–12 times, keeping the palms as flat as
possible on the foot. Hold the foot again to finish.

THUMB KNEADING MOVEMENT 2   To ease out any tension or tightness gently rub the sole and the surface of the foot with the thumbs, using
small circles. First rub down between the tendons on top, then work
across the sole. Rub your thumbs around the bones on the ankle joint.

PALM KNEADING MOVEMENT 3   Holding the foot with one hand,
use the palm of the other hand to work over the sole. Then work the palm
over the top and sides of the foot.

STROKING MOVEMENT 4   Using the flat of the hands, slowly and
rhythmically rub the upper surface of the foot with one hand and the sole
with the other as at the beginning of the massage. Repeat 10–12 times.

HOLDING MOVEMENT 5   Hold the foot for 30 seconds and then cover
it with the towel.

FINISH   Repeat these movements on the other foot, then hold both
covered feet gently for another 30 seconds to finish off the sequence.

- Do not put heavy pressure on bony areas.
- Do not put heavy pressure on organs (heart, abdomen, small of back).
- Stop immediately if massage causes pain (unless it feels like therapeutic pain).
- Do not massage where there is new scar tissue, nor in cases of cancer.
- Do not massage where there are any circulatory problems, asthma, epilepsy, severe or chronic back pain, long-term injury, or skin infections.

Self-help

Self-massage can be useful when there is no one else around. For headaches, massage the temples with circular movements, using the fingertips. Using a shampooing motion on the hair can also relieve tension and tightness in the head. End by gently pulling strands of hair to improve the circulation to the scalp.

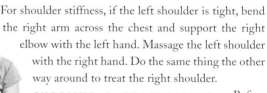

Massaging your shoulders is an effective way to relieve stiffness.

Relieve a head-ache by massaging your temples.

For shoulder stiffness, if the left shoulder is tight, bend the right arm across the chest and support the right elbow with the left hand. Massage the left shoulder with the right hand. Do the same thing the other way around to treat the right shoulder.

CHOOSING A PRACTITIONER Before going for a massage, be sure that you ask about the training, qualifications, and experience of the practitioner.

Is a massage compatible with conventional medicine?
In general, yes. If you have a serious health problem, you should check with your doctor first.

Is a practitioner necessary?
For an effective therapeutic massage you need a qualified practitioner, but a simple massage with a partner can be relaxing and enjoyable.

Shiatsu

Shiatsu (from the Japanese "shi," meaning finger, and "atsu," pressure) has its theoretical and practical roots in the East. A Shiatsu practitioner diagnoses and treats his or her client using energy pathways (meridians) of the body, and points (tsubos).

In China and Japan until the late 19th century, gaining competence in bodywork was a prerequisite for the qualification of every physician. Shiatsu administered by friends and family for relaxation and the relief of minor ailments has also successfully been used in the home.

With evolving communications between East and West, different medical modalities (approaches) are being explored and appreciated and Shiatsu is now used increasingly in the West. Shiatsu makes use of traditional Chinese medicine and the "S-element" and meridian systems to promote healing. During the 20th century, the modern understanding of anatomy, physiology, and psychology have also been incorporated into the practice of Shiatsu.

In Shiatsu, pressure is applied along the meridians (energy channels) to treat health problems.

WILL IT HELP?

• Many conditions can be treated successfully with Shiatsu, including functional disturbances of the inner organs, stress-related symptoms, migraines, muscle pain in the neck and back, arthritis, gynecological conditions, exhaustion, and general debility. Shiatsu is helpful during pregnancy. It supports well-being and can be used as a long-term preventive treatment.

BENEFITS

• Treats stress, migraines, muscular pain, and arthritis.
• Is beneficial during pregnancy.
• Complements Western medicine by providing the physical and psychological support that increasingly overburdened hospitals cannot always offer.
• Aids speedy recovery from illness.
• Can provide help during difficult periods in life, such as relationship breakdowns or redundancy.
• Helps to maintain general well-being.

CAUTION

• Seek medical advice before undergoing Shiatsu if you are suffering from a serious medical condition.
• Some conditions are contra-indicated, namely: acute infections, recent operations and injuries, and severe psychoses.
• Particular care needs to be taken working with clients with cancer, thrombosis, and osteoporosis.
• The energetic effect of Shiatsu may be limited with alcoholics, drug addicts, and those on strong medication.

Key principles

The well-being of a person physically, emotionally, and spiritually depends on the distribution and flow of energy ("ki" in Japanese, "chi" in Chinese). This is affected by energetic inheritance, emotions, injury, infection, lifestyle, and the weather. A Shiatsu practitioner works using various methods, from subtle, supportive contact and holding, to more dynamic pressure and stretching. Deficient energy can be tonified and excess or stagnant energy dispersed or reduced. Muscles, joints, blood, and fluids are influenced, and circulation, flexibility, and vitality increased. Shiatsu can be done with the recipient sitting or lying down. No equipment is necessary.

Shiatsu practitioners work predominantly with their hands. The fundamental principle involves diagnosing and treating the kyo (empty) and jitsu (full) meridians in the body. The aim of Shiatsu is to support the client's strengths, release tensions, and activate his or her regenerative power. In Shiatsu, a cohesive diagnostic structure is combined with the connection and sensitivity that physical touch enables. The practitioner looks not only at the presenting condition but also, if the client is ill, at the underlying cause. In Eastern medicine the delineation between sickness and health that exists in Western medicine is less strict. Indeed "sickness" may be a healthy response to certain phenomena in an individual's life.

Different forms

The various forms of Shiatsu are similar in their fundamental principles, but their methods vary. Some place the emphasis on the working of individual points, others on links between food and the meridian system, yet others on the influence of psychological factors on the meridian system.

PRACTITIONER-LED: WHAT TO EXPECT Shiatsu is mainly done as the client lies, clothed, on a supportive mat on the floor. A session usually lasts one hour, but the duration and frequency of treatment will vary from person to person, as will the total number of sessions.

Shiatsu begins with a consultation about your health and treatment aims. Treatment involves the application of pressure along the meridian lines with attention to certain points. At the end, time is given for the client to be still and reflect. After this, there may be a brief discussion between client and practitioner on the treatment, and recommendations may be made about diet, exercises, and lifestyle.

Treatment usually leaves a feeling of calm and well-being and of being more in touch with one's body, healing capacity, and the world around, and often results in renewed vigor and clarity of mind.

DIAGNOSIS In Shiatsu four methods of diagnosing are used: observation, listening to the sound of voice, listening to the (actual) words that are being said, and touching.

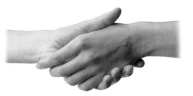

A simple handshake gives us an impression of the other person. Shiatsu takes this touch diagnosis further.

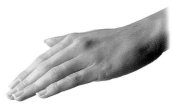

Human touch itself is a great healer, providing comfort to the recipient, as well as the other benefits of Shiatsu.

Self-Shiatsu (known as "Do-in") can be done on the parts of the body that can be reached easily—the face is an obvious choice.

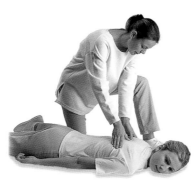

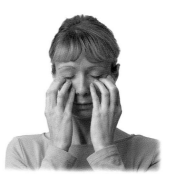

The practitioner uses her body weight to apply pressure during a Shiatsu massage, helping the recipient to relax.

 Is Shiatsu compatible with conventional medicine?
Yes, although if you are taking strong medication the full energizing effect of Shiatsu may not be felt.

 Is a practitioner necessary?
Shiatsu is used as a home remedy but accurate diagnostic skills are generally achieved through professional training. It is well to remember, however, that Shiatsu is not merely a technique-oriented therapy. The qualities of sincerity, simplicity, and being nonjudgmental are essential in a practitioner.

Aromatherapy

The use of perfumed plants is intimately linked to the develop-ment of medicine and in this way the history of aromatherapy dates back to the early civilizations of the Mesopotamian area and the East. Chaldeans, Babylonians, the pharaohs and queens of Egypt, and the cultures of Ancient Greece, Persia, Rome, and India all partook of its benefits, with no division seemingly being made between the pleasure and the medicinal benefits of plant perfumes. The essential oils of aromatherapy eventually moved into the royal houses of Europe around the 16th century. It was only in the 1960s, however, that aromatherapy as we know it today was developed, largely through the work of Marguerite Maury. It is now recognized as a useful complementary medicine, invaluable in preventive treatment.

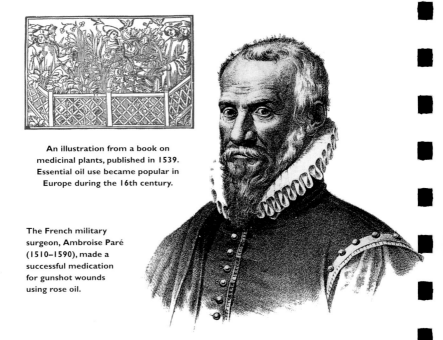

An illustration from a book on medicinal plants, published in 1539. Essential oil use became popular in Europe during the 16th century.

The French military surgeon, Ambroise Paré (1510–1590), made a successful medication for gunshot wounds using rose oil.

WILL IT HELP?

- Aromatherapy uses plant essences chiefly to enhance the beneficial effects of massage, both physiologically and mentally, but also in other forms of treatment.
- Specific essential oils can help in such conditions as bronchitis, rheumatism, genitourinary problems, and premenstrual syndrome.
- Aromatherapy massage boosts the immune system and has a settling effect.
- Back pain, headaches, migraines, neuralgias and depression will all respond to treatment with the right essential oils.
- The therapy is especially good as preventive treatment, through dealing with the effects of stress, now acknowledged to be involved in many cases of illness and disease.

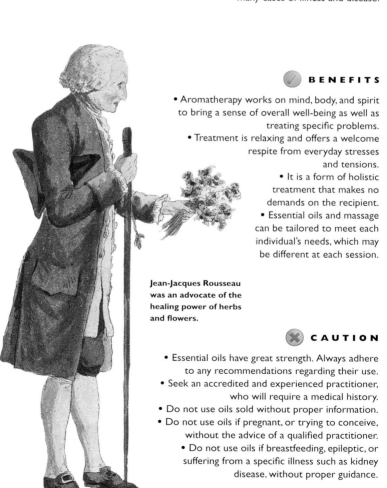

BENEFITS

- Aromatherapy works on mind, body, and spirit to bring a sense of overall well-being as well as treating specific problems.
- Treatment is relaxing and offers a welcome respite from everyday stresses and tensions.
- It is a form of holistic treatment that makes no demands on the recipient.
- Essential oils and massage can be tailored to meet each individual's needs, which may be different at each session.

Jean-Jacques Rousseau was an advocate of the healing power of herbs and flowers.

CAUTION

- Essential oils have great strength. Always adhere to any recommendations regarding their use.
- Seek an accredited and experienced practitioner, who will require a medical history.
- Do not use oils sold without proper information.
- Do not use oils if pregnant, or trying to conceive, without the advice of a qualified practitioner.
- Do not use oils if breastfeeding, epileptic, or suffering from a specific illness such as kidney disease, without proper guidance.

Natural therapy

Aromatherapy is a completely natural form of treatment, in both the substances it uses and the way in which they are administered. Essential oils are unadulterated oils extracted from flowers, stems, roots, leaves, seeds, or bark of plants. Their biologically active compounds contain vital elements that affect the body systems in a variety of ways and act as catalysts in healing. Oils are used in complementary medicine both preventively and in treatment of specific conditions, but one of their advantages is that they can also be used easily at home in a number of ways. Because of their strength essential oils are used diluted in a bland carrier oil, and it is inadvisable to apply undiluted oils directly to the skin.

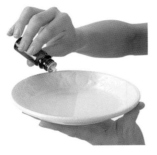 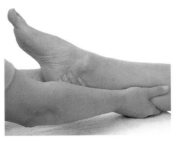

Essential oils must always be diluted in a carrier, such as sweet almond oil, light coconut oil, or jojoba oil.

Aromatherapy massage employs various techniques, including stroking, kneading, and pummeling movements.

Professional treatment

In professional aromatherapy the oils are used mainly in massage treatment. A massage with essential oils encourages the oils to be absorbed by the skin and into the circulatory system while the molecules are also absorbed into the respiratory system through the breath. At the same time the scent of the oils has an effect on the mind. Oils can be stimulating, calming, or balancing at a mental level, and have similar effects on the body. Specific oils can stimulate particular systems of the body, simultaneously acting beneficially on other functions. For example, rosemary (*Rosmarinus officinalis*) has a positive effect on the circulation and can help to treat hypotension; it is also an aid to digestion, a stimulant to the immune system, and a restorative that helps to concentrate the mind. Essential oils may be used clinically by trained clinical therapists or other medical professionals. In such cases they may be administered orally or in other carefully controlled ways, for the treatment of specific clinical problems.

Using oils at home

In home use, essential oils can be enjoyed for their scent alone, or added to skin creams and body and scalp lotions. Used in vaporizers they impart their volatile ingredients to the air, either simply to give a pleasant scent to the room. Or, they can be used to disinfect a sickroom, alleviate breathing problems, and even to keep insects at bay. Through steam inhalation anti-septic oils can help to decongest blocked noses and sinuses, and introduce their therapeutic properties into the respiratory system. They can also be applied to pillows and handkerchiefs for inhalation.

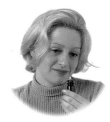

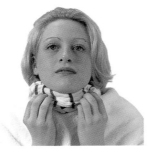

Make a hot compress by soaking a cloth in 17 fl oz (500ml) water, to which 5 or 6 drops of essential oil have been added.

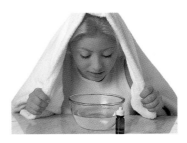

Inhaling steam from aromatherapy oils diluted in hot water helps to relieve congestion.

Beauty therapy

Nowadays a huge range of toiletries, from soaps, bath additives, shampoos, and hair-care products, to face and body oils, creams, and lotions, claim to be part of aromatherapy. Unless the labeling specifically states that only pure essential oils are used it is likely that synthetic scents are used in the product. However, base creams, lotions, gels, and shampoos to which essential oils of your choice can be added, can be purchased or even made at home.

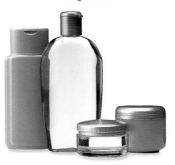

Add essential oils to base cream, oil, gel, and shampoo to create tailor-made products.

NAME	PROPERTIES
CHAMOMILE German, Roman (*Matricaria recutica, Anthemis nobilis*)	Analgesic, sedative; reduces fever; bactericidal; eases spasm; assists menstruation
EUCALYPTUS (*Eucalyptus globulus*)	Analgesic, antineuralgic; antiseptic; acts against parasites; antiviral, expectorant; balsamic (soothing)
FRANKINCENSE (*Boswellia carteri*)	Nerve tonic, sedative (slows and deepens breathing); antiseptic, immune stimulant, expectorant; vulnery, cicatrisant; encourages growth of skin cells; anti-inflammatory, astringent; carminative; assists menstruation, genitourinary tonic
JUNIPER (*Juniperus communis*)	Nerve tonic, sedative; antiseptic; cicatrisant, skin toner; detoxifying in bloodstream and digestive system; rubefacient; diuretic, antiseptic; tonic, especially of genitourinary system
LAVENDER, TRUE (*Lavandula angustifolia*)	Analgesic, nerve tonic, sedative, antidepressant; antitoxic, anti-infectious, also a deodorant; carminative; rubefacient; insecticide
PEPPERMINT (*Mentha piperita*)	Analgesic, (local) anesthetic, stimulant; antiseptic, expectorant, stimulant; digestive aid, tonic
ROSE (*Rosa centifolia/damascena*)	Antidepressant, sedative; hemostatic (controls bleeding), antiseptic; cicatrisant, astringent; circulatory tonic; detoxicant, laxative; tonic
ROSEMARY (*Rosmarinus officinalis*)	Analgesic, stimulant, cephalic (mental tonic); astringent, regulates seborrhea; cordial tonic; antirheumatic; acts against parasites; antimicrobial, antioxidant; liver tonic and digestive
SAGE, CLARY (*Salvia sclarea*)	Anticonvulsive, antidepressant, euphoric, antispasmodic, sedative; antiseptic; bactericidal, also a good deodorant; astringent; digestive; tonic
VETIVERT (*Vetiveria zizanoides*)	Antiseptic; rubefacient; sedative, tonic, makes a deeply grounding relaxant; antitoxic, encourages production of red blood corpuscles, blood cleanser; stimulant to circulatory system

TREATS

CAUTIONS

Nervous tension, insomnia, headache, stress; influenza, infection; burns, cuts; acne, allergies, rashes; indigestion, colic, nausea, arthritis, rheumatism, pain; dysmenorrhea (scanty periods), menorrhagia (heavy periods)

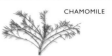

CHAMOMILE

Neuralgia, debility, headaches; skin eruptions, herpes, bites; parasites, scabies; coughs, phlegm, colds, throat infections; rheumatic conditions; muscular aches and pains

EUCALYPTUS

Asthma, bronchitis, anxiety, panic, nervous tension, stress; coughs, colds, influenza, laryngitis; wounds, sores, blemishes, scars; wrinkles, dry or aging skin; skin care; menstrual problems, leukorrhea, cystitis

FRANKINCENSE

Stress conditions; infections, colds, influenza; wounds; cellulite, circulatory problems, obesity, gout; arthritis, rheumatism; cystitis, edema; leukorrhea, menstrual problems

JUNIPER
Overuse can be harmful to the kidneys

Stress, premenstrual syndrome, depression, insomnia, hypertension; skin eruptions and inflammation, infection, especially respiratory infections; burns, rashes; intestinal gas; muscular aches and pains

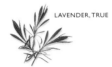

LAVENDER, TRUE

Mental fatigue, fainting, headache, stress; phlegm, colds, fevers, influenza, acne, congested skin; dyspepsia, liver and bile disorders, nausea

PEPPERMINT

Depression, frigidity, impotence, insomnia, premenstrual syndrome; broken capillaries, herpes, eczema, wounds, sensitive skin, wrinkles; anxiety; liver congestion, nausea

ROSE
Do not use in acute conditions without professional medical advice

Debility, mental exhaustion, poor concentration, headache; dandruff, scalp conditions; poor circulation and related problems; muscular pain, gout, rheumatism; lice, scabies; colds, influenza, intestinal infections, colitis

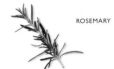

ROSEMARY

Hyper-reactions, depression, nervous tension, stress-related disorders, migraines, muscle aches and pains, asthma; acne, boils, dandruff; infections; oily skin and hair; digestive system, gas problems; nervous system, female reproductive system

SAGE, CLARY
Should not be used with alcohol, which increases its euphoria-inducing and sedative effects and can cause nausea

Oily skin, cuts and wounds; muscular aches and pains, arthritis, rheumatism, sprains and stiffness; debility, depression, insomnia, tension

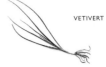

VETIVERT

Mind and body therapy

Essential oils have antiseptic, fungicidal, and anti-inflammatory properties that can help the immune system to resist and fight infection and treat
all manner of skin problems, such as acne, boils, abscesses, rashes (including herpes), stretch marks, scars, bruising, and inflammation. Oils can also
alleviate burns, disinfect and help to heal cuts, chapped or cracked skin,
and treat fungal infections such as athlete's foot, dandruff, ringworm, and
lice. They can be applied in the form of proprietary or homemade preparations, or diluted in carrier oils. Some oils are effective in promoting
healthy circulation and dealing with chilblains and varicose veins, while
others actively help rheumatic joints and muscular pain. Healing or calming oils can also be added to hot or cold compresses to give extra benefit
when these are used. Diluted essential oils can be used in the bath for their
therapeutic value as well as their pleasant scent.

In general, aromatherapy, whether practitioner- or self-administered,
can help to release tension and anxiety, deal with shock, uplift the spirits,
and promote a new sense of balance. Back pain,
sciatica, headaches, migraines, neuralgia, and
depression will all respond to
treatment with the right
essential oils.

All oils should be diluted before
use and used externally only,
unless otherwise instructed by
a qualified practitioner. They
can be massaged into the skin,
used in the bath, or inhaled.

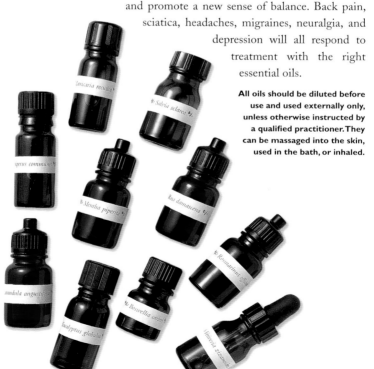

OILS FOR USE AT HOME   Some essential oils are effective in promoting circulation, helping to deal with circulatory complaints such as chilblains and varicose veins. Many essential oils are active detoxicants or have anti-inflammatory effects, helping rheumatic joint conditions and reducing muscular pain. Others are adept at aiding the respiratory system to fight or avert the common cold, influenza and ancillary ailments, reliev-

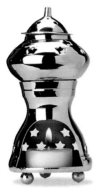

ing chills, coughs, laryngitis, hoarseness, congestion, and conditions such as bronchitis and asthma. Many oils are multifaceted in their effects and work on mind and spirit as well as body.

Oil burners can be used to disperse the effects of essential oils throughout a room. Always read the instructions before using oils in a burner and keep them away from children.

Insomnia

Insomnia causes the body to be run-down and can lead to a number of unpleasant conditions. A healthy diet and sensible daily exercise encourage good sleep, as do eating early in the evening, and unwinding and relaxing before going to bed. Lavender essential oil can also help. Use the oil to vaporize the bedroom before going to bed or sprinkle a few drops on the pillow and bottom sheet, so that you can breathe in its sedative scent.

For people who sleep restlessly, rose oil can help. Put two drops of the oil onto a small cotton ball, tape it to the cuplike cartilage of the upper external ear, and leave it overnight. This method is also suitable for older children.

For a good night's sleep rose oil will help restless sleepers while lavender oil can help insomniacs.

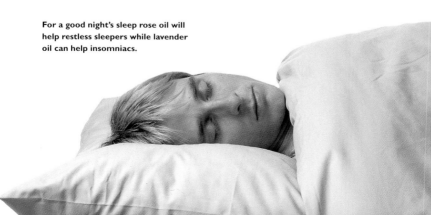

Aromatherapy massage

A massage is a natural formalization of the primitive instinct to rub the body when it has been hurt. Neuromuscular tension in any part of the body, usually caused by mental stress, can result in serious illnesses and disease, and can be greatly alleviated by a massage. The essential oils used in aromatherapy enhance the effect.

Aromatherapy massage is a form of herbalism practiced directly on the body, advantageously bypassing the digestive tract, and has the ability to stimulate organs and functions such as circulation, skin, muscles, and joints, and the whole nervous system. It extends its remedial influence to the respiratory, genitourinary, endocrine, and lymphatic systems, as well as bolstering the body's immune defenses. A relaxing aromatherapy massage with essential oils helps to enhance good health and a sense of well-being of body, mind, and spirit.

HEAD-AND-FACE MASSAGE   A head-and-face massage is relaxing and comforting. Use 2 tsp (10ml) of a carrier oil such as light coconut or sweet almond oil and three to four drops of the essential oil of your choice.

1 Using fingertips, with light circular movements, release stress and stimulate the forehead's circulation at least three times.

2 Working in panels from the base of the back of the neck and over the head to the forehead, release tension and activate circulation using firmer tiny circular movements with fingertips and thumbs.

3 Using the fingertips, make a series of long, gentle, stroking movements with alternate hands from the base of the neck up to the jawline. Repeat several times.

It's quite possible to give yourself a comforting and relaxing head and face massage to relieve tension and stress.

4 Using the second and third fingertips of both hands simultaneously, with firm pressure, work up from the chin past the nasomental lines up to the hairline. Repeat three times.

5 Using the second and third fingertips of both hands simultaneously, with firm pressure, move either side of the chin to the sides of the nose and describe a triangle outward under the cheekbones to the ears. Repeat three times.

6 In the same way, work from the base of the chin to describe the oval of the outer limits of the face, going past the ears upward, to meet at the center of the hairline. Repeat three times.

7 With thumbs drawn outward, use splayed, stroking, descending outward movements from the hairline over the forehead, under the cheekbones to the ears. Use fingertips in a lightly vibrating drumming movement, continuing on either sides of the upper jawbone to mid-point of chin. Repeat three times.

8 Finally, using outer sides of thumbs, stroke firmly in a downward direction to increase lymphatic drainage and help eliminate waste matter. Repeat three times.

Anxiety patch

Butterflies in the stomach at interviews or nerves before an examination may proceed from thought associations. On such occasions our sense of smell and the direct pathway that smelling opens to the brain, together with the uptake through the skin of a calming essential oil, can come to the rescue, helping to reduce anxiety, tension, and panic. Rose oil is particularly therapeutic in such circumstances.

Is aromatherapy compatible with conventional medicine?
Essential oils will not interfere with any medical treatment. and will help to produce a positive sense of well-being.

Is a practitioner necessary?
A practitioner is not required for many simple uses of essential oils and gentle oils such as lavender and chamomile. For full aromatherapy treatments it is essential to seek the advice and supervision of a qualified and registered professional aromatherapist.

Are oils safe?
All information regarding any essential oil should be read and followed.

Reflexology

Reflexology is one of the most popular complementary therapies available today. It is simple, safe, and very effective: the patient does not need to undress and the therapist uses only the hands to give a treatment. Another advantage is that it is ideally suited for use in conjunction with orthodox medicine. It is a noninvasive treatment, cooperating with the body's own healing processes to induce a state of balance and well-being. As a true complementary medicine it can also help the body to counteract the side effects of drugs or other treatment and is very valuable in aiding recovery after illness, operations, or fractures.

What is reflexology?

Reflexology is based on the concept that all parts of the body are connected by energy pathways, which end in the feet, the hands and the head. "Reflex" in the context of "reflexology" means the reflection of all the organs, systems, and structures of the body onto the feet or hands, and reflexology is the practice of working over these reflexes in a precise and systematic way.

The practitioner, by applying controlled pressure with the thumbs or fingers to the reflex areas, stimulates the body to achieve its own state of equilibrium and good health. Pressure on the reflexes affects an organ or region of the body and also influences the relationship between different functions, processes, and parts.

History of reflexology

The concept of stimulating the body's healing energies by using pressure points on the feet is not new. It has appeared in many different cultures around the world and throughout history. Earliest traces have been found from more than 5,000 years ago in China, Japan, and Egypt. It spread to Europe in the Dark Ages and forms of "pressure point" therapy were used in the Middle Ages by both peasants and the aristocracy. The therapy was rediscovered in the late 1890s by a Dr. William Fitzgerald and introduced into the United States as "reflexology."

WILL IT HELP?

• Reflexology is a helpful and relaxing complementary therapy that can be a useful adjunct in the treatment—whether conventional or alternative—of many health problems. Children and babies as well as adults can benefit from this treatment. In particular the following conditions have shown improvement: sinusitis, asthma, migraines, depression, muscular and skeletal disorders, menstrual problems, hypertension, bowel disorders. It has also helped small babies with colic, and women with pregnancy-related problems

The positions of the reflex areas on the feet correspond closely to the relative positions of the organs, glands, or structures of the body itself

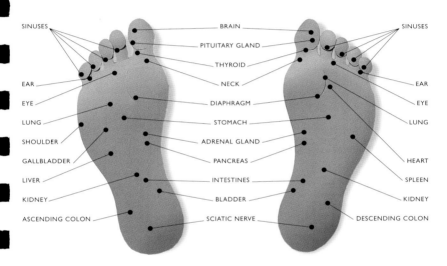

 BENEFITS

• Reflexology is simple and safe.
• Treatment is relaxing and often leads to a general improvement in well-being.

 CAUTION

• Reflexology is an extremely safe therapy and there are few contraindications. However, there are some circumstances in which care should be taken. Children are very sensitive and responsive, so short, light treatments are recommended. Certain reflexes should not be stimulated during early pregnancy, although reflexology is very effective for reducing morning sickness, high blood pressure, and back pain. Special treatment plans may be needed for clients taking drugs that may affect the body's natural homeostasis, such as immunosuppressants, steroids, fertility treatment, or hormone replacement therapy, or if a pacemaker has been fitted or if there has been a recent organ transplant.

Reflexology today

Eunice Ingham, an American physician, developed Fitzgerald's theories and produced a comprehensive chart that mapped all the body's reflexes onto the feet. As new schools were set up, some kept to Ingham's original method while others developed new techniques. Because of the evolving, dynamic nature of the therapy there is now some diversity between schools, both in views taken on the exact location of some of the reflexes and in the method of treatment. Such differences fall within the basic principles of reflexology and do not detract from its effectiveness.

How does reflexology work?

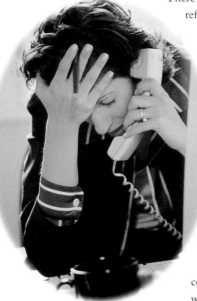

There are several theories as to how reflexology works. The traditional belief is that energy, or "life force," flows through channels in the body. When these channels become blocked or the energy flow depleted, parts of the body are starved of this energy, becoming dis-eased. Reflexology clears the channels and restores the free flow of vital energy. A modern theory is that it works through the nervous system. There are more than 70,000 nerve endings in the feet, which connect via the spinal cord to all parts of the body. By working on the nerve endings reflexology may stimulate the nervous system to normal, healthy functioning. Other theories include interaction with the body's electro-magnetic fields; working with the body's natural vibrations and healing potential; and the breaking down of waste deposits collected in the feet.

Sometimes stress seems to hurl itself from all corners of our lives. It is important to take steps to prevent it from developing into illness.

WHAT CONDITIONS CAN BE HELPED? Reflexology is a holistic therapy recognizing every individual's capacity for self-healing. Practitioners do not treat problems—they treat people. Reflexologists do not claim to cure diseases and reflexology is not a substitute for orthodox medical treatment. It has proved very beneficial for a wide range of chronic and acute conditions, however, and especially for stress-related problems, which lie at the root of so many modern illnesses.

Reflexology helps to release physical tension and mental strain, so allowing the body's own healing potential to restore health and well-being on all levels. Many practitioners have reported that clients with problems such as sinusitis, asthma, migraines, depression, muscular and skeletal disorders, menstrual problems, hypertension, and bowel disorders have benefited from treatment. Reflexology can also help small babies with colic, maintain athletes in peak condition, and bring peace to the dying.

GOING FOR A TREATMENT

One of the advantages of reflexology is that the whole body can be treated through the feet (or sometimes the hands), so the client only has to take off their shoes and socks. For each person the application and effect of the therapy is unique and the experienced practitioner will tailor treatment to each individual.

A treatment session usually lasts for about one hour. Although a single session helps to reduce tension, several treatments may be needed before the full benefits are felt, particularly if problems are deep-seated. The number of sessions and their frequency will depend on individual requirements, and the

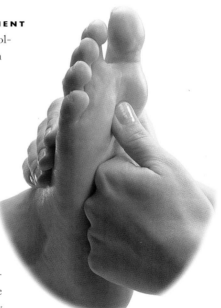

Reflexology has been found beneficial for stress-related problems. The feet take a pounding every day and as the practitioner works there is the additional benefit of deep relaxation that reflexology brings.

qualified reflexologist will devise an appropriate treatment plan with the client. After treatment there may be a temporary reaction as the body readjusts or releases toxins. This could be a feeling of well-being, of relaxation, or perhaps a little lethargy, a sensation of being "off color," or even weepiness. Such feelings are short-lived and part of the healing process.

Because relaxation is one of the main benefits of reflexology it is best to let someone else work on your feet or hands. Some self-help techniques, however, can be used to release tension in stressful circumstances. For most people hands are more accessible than feet and it is usually more appropriate to work on your own hands. It is also far less noticeable when giving a self-help treatment in public.

1 Before starting, sit quietly for a few moments and breathe deeply. Relax your shoulders, rest your hands in your lap, and place both feet on the ground. The diaphragm and solar plexus are areas most affected by tension and these are the reflexes to work on first of all.

2 To release tension, place the thumb of one hand into the palm of the other and gently press upward into the space between the knuckles of the index and middle fingers.

3 At the same time take a deep breath in and then breathe out slowly, letting shoulders, arms, and stomach relax as the pressure of the thumb is maintained for about ten seconds. The hand being "worked" should be relaxed and curl over the thumb.

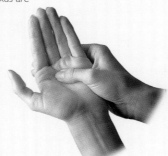

Self-help techniques can be used on the hands, so that you can have treatment wherever you are.

4 Repeat three or four times on each palm, and follow with a circular massage movement all over the palms of both hands.

5 Then gently squeeze each finger in turn, rotate the knuckle, stretch the finger and slide your hand off.

The same techniques can be used on the feet, and rotating the toes and ankle joints helps to release tension in the neck and back.

 Is this therapy compatible with conventional medicine?
Reflexology can help as an adjunct to the conventional treatment of many conditions, although some types of drugs will lessen its effects.

 Is a practitioner necessary?
A practitioner is recommended.

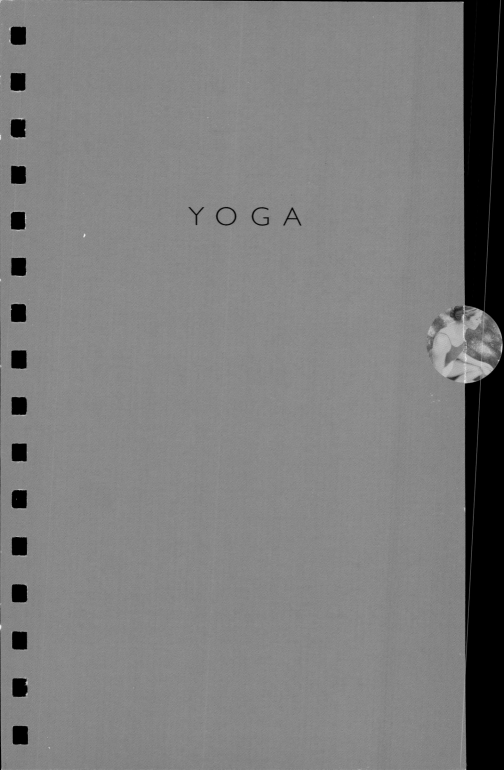

Y O G A

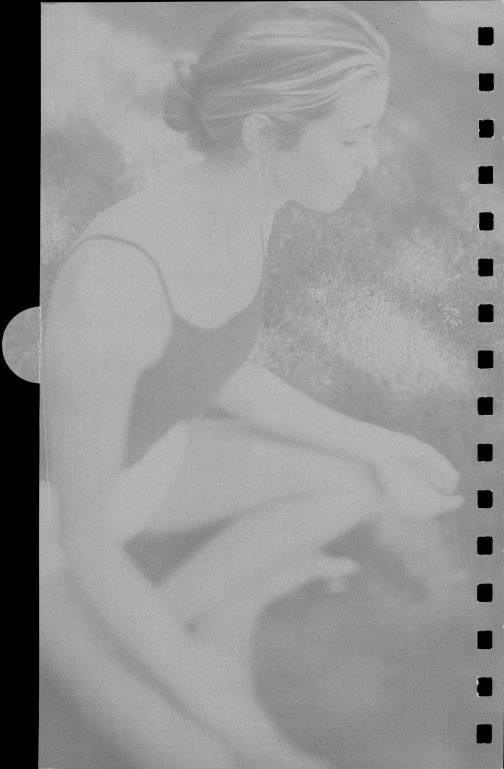

Although yoga is an Eastern-based therapy it has long been popular in the West. In fact, so many people have discovered the therapeutic joys of yoga that it barely qualifies as an "alternative" activity any longer. Like all the best therapies, yoga can be practiced by people of any age; and is suitable for pregnant women. Because it is intended to promote suppleness and balance instead of muscular fitness it does not demand a high level of fitness as a prerequisite. There are many forms of yoga, a few of them far beyond the average person, but most of which can be learned gradually, at an individual's own pace. A practitioner is essential for any form of yoga. No one should practice yoga without having followed at least a basic course first.

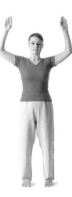

Yoga

Although yoga as practiced in the West is thought of as being primarily a series of stretching exercises and postures that develop calm of mind and flexibility of body, the ultimate goals of yoga are to meditate and to raise the mind above the difficulties of life. In Ancient times yoga was pure meditation, but to prepare body and mind for meditation yoga masters devised a series of physical postures known as asanas. Accompanied by correct yogic breathing, the asanas stimulate the nervous system, while the joints and muscles become more flexible and the mind and body relax. All yoga exercises are interspersed with moments of relaxation and stillness.

The Buddha was one of the first yogis and is often shown sitting in the Lotus position.

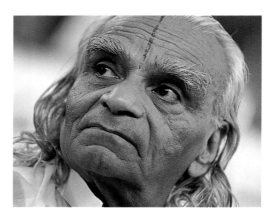

B.K.S. Iyengar is probably the most famous yoga teacher of the 20th century, and was instrumental in introducing this Indian therapy to the Western world.

WILL IT HELP?

• Yoga is a holistic therapy that exercises the body and calms the mind. Because it emphasizes correct posture and breathing combined with stretching exercises, it promotes general good health through improved circulation and blood pressure.
• It has been found to have a beneficial effect on back pain, RSI and MS. It also helps to prevent osteoporosis by building bone density, and relieves the problems caused by overuse of joints and limbs.

 CAUTION

• Yoga must be practiced gently with correct breathing and properly prepared muscles. Anyone with a medical condition including heart or back problems, dizziness, or high blood pressure should seek medical advice before starting.

 BENEFITS

• Daily yoga practice promotes the body's healthy maintenance through improved oxygen and blood supply.
• It has been found to be very beneficial as a means of relieving stress and tension through exercise and relaxation.
• Yoga also improves suppleness, strength, stamina, digestion, concentration, and relaxation and can alleviate hyperventilation and asthma.

The goal of calm

Preparation is an important part of yoga training, since both the mind and the body need to be receptive before attempting the asanas. Each yoga session begins with stretching exercises that flex the body, while the focus of the mind is on tranquillity. The asanas, followed by relaxation, work on all parts of an individual's personal life to promote health and well-being, making yoga a holistic therapy with both physical and spiritual aspects. Primarily a preventive therapy, yoga helps to convert anger and frustration into calm and self-control.

Yoga also has an ethical dimension. The yoga masters who expanded the philosophy and practice of yoga over the centuries developed an approach to life based on nonviolence and integrity. Their belief that both perpetrator and recipient are damaged by harmful actions remains a key principle of yoga today.

The goal of calm makes yoga an especially appropriate therapy for counteracting the pressures of modern life. Students can combine the teachings of past yoga masters with today's scientific research. Many illnesses are now known to be stress-related, and yoga can help to counteract stress, as well as the ill-effects of a lack of exercise. The ability to control the mind and body at will that yoga fosters can lower blood pressure, ease stress, and recover a sense of self that is often lost among the demands of modern living.

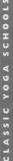

CLASSIC YOGA SCHOOLS

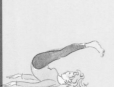

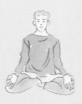

Hatha yoga
Helps students to overcome the turmoil of life today and links the teaching of the Ancient yoga masters with modern practice.

Raja yoga
Meditation is the basis of raja yoga and students follow stages of deep meditation. Many statues of the Buddha show him practicing raja yoga.

Karma yoga
Followers of karma yoga live for the moment, opening their minds to allow things to happen. In this state the right and selfless action becomes clear.

The schools of yoga

Yoga masters have always understood that there are many ways to carry out the quest for inner peace and understanding. Over the centuries, several schools of yoga have sprung up, and new ones continue to develop. The six main classic schools of yoga use different methods to achieve the same aim. These range from the prolonged meditation of raja yoga, to karma yoga, which teaches that by being quiet and opening up to intuition, we will know what action to take to help others. Jnana yoga revolves around study of the ancient yoga texts, while bhakti yoga focuses on worship of a deity. Mantra yoga raises consciousness through the chanting of phrases, words, and sounds known as mantras.

The sixth school, hatha yoga, is the form most commonly practiced in the West: it teaches control of the mind through asana (physical postures), pranayama (breath control), and deep relaxation. It emerged about 1,000 years ago as an introductory form of yoga to help beginners learn control over body and mind in preparation for the deeper stage of meditation.

The 20th century saw the development of other forms of yoga. Iyengar yoga is named after B.K.S. Iyengar who, in the 1950s, created a more gymnastic approach, with less emphasis on breathing and meditation. Ashtanga yoga, an ancient form rediscovered in the 1930s, helps the body to shed toxins and realign the skeletal structure. Viniyoga, another ancient form, emphasizes individual needs and very gradual progression.

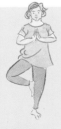

Bhakti yoga
Followers of bhakti yoga reach self-awareness through worship. A personal yoga, it suits those who follow a religion or who are naturally spiritual.

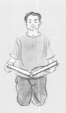

Jnana yoga
Students of the jnana (pronounced "gyana") school seek answers to life's great questions by reading and discussing the classic yoga texts.

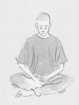

Mantra yoga
Chanting mantras is associated with Tibetan monks, who practice this form of yoga. Chanting aids concentration and the attainment of higher states of consciousness.

Fitting yoga into your life

Yoga is a constant learning process and for this reason it is better to join a class taught by a qualified teacher. Simple exercises can be practiced at home, and the key to success is commitment to regular sessions. For maximum benefit yoga organizations recommend at least 20 minutes a day in a calm space where you will not be disturbed.

POSTURE AND BREATHING Good posture and effective breathing lead to high energy levels, relaxed muscles, and peace of mind and are fundamental to yoga. The yoga asanas gradually correct faulty posture and breathing. Because many of the asanas are done sitting on the floor, sitting correctly is vital if they are to be effective.

When you are sitting correctly, your shoulders will be straight, with head, neck, and back upright. In this position the muscles align the bones correctly, allowing easy movement of the diaphragm, which stimulates the body's neuroelectrical system and leads to better circulation.

Breathing is an automatic function, but breathing correctly has great benefits in terms of energy levels and relaxation. Yoga places great importance on pranayama—breath control—and all hatha yoga exercises and asanas are accompanied by pranayama. Over time, the exercises and asanas give students an awareness of their breathing patterns and enable them to modify the way in which they breathe, benefiting both mind and body.

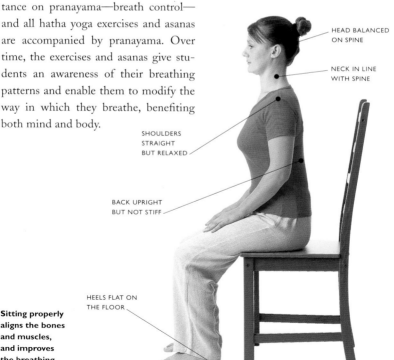

HEAD BALANCED ON SPINE

NECK IN LINE WITH SPINE

SHOULDERS STRAIGHT BUT RELAXED

BACK UPRIGHT BUT NOT STIFF

HEELS FLAT ON THE FLOOR

Sitting properly aligns the bones and muscles, and improves the breathing.

THE POSTURE TEST   Test your sitting posture with a paper cup. While you sit at work, put an empty cup upside down on the crown of your head and try to keep it there. It will keep falling off until you move into a better posture. You will feel the benefits—better breathing and concentration—once you can keep the cup in place for about five minutes.

STANDING POSTURE   Balancing the body is extremely important in yoga. You can check your posture using this simple method.

1 Stand against a wall, as erect as you can. Your head and heels should be half and inch (1.5cm) away from the wall. Adjust your posture if they are not.

2 Walk around the room, then try to return to the same posture against the wall. Repeat the exercise until your posture ensures that your head and heels are always the same distance from the wall when you return to it.

PLANNING A YOGA PROGRAM   There is no need to have a set time of day or duration for the program, but practice must be regular: a daily session (as little as 20 minutes a day is beneficial), or a longer weekly session, is essential.

When planning your program, keep an overview to make sure that no part of the body is ignored. Working on the back is a good place to begin, since flexibility of the spine will help you to perform the other asanas. You can work on the back in one session, and the neck and shoulders in another. Asanas can be performed in any order, but you should choose asanas that provide a balanced exercise for the body. Balance and counterbalance are important, so you should always follow forward bends with backward bends. You should also allow time for relaxation between exercises.

KEY ELEMENTS OF A PROGRAM

Timings are for a 90-minute session but can be adapted to fit the time available.

1 Warm-up stretches: 10 minutes
2 Relaxation: 1 minute
3 Breathing: 10 minutes
4 Asana sequences: 50 minutes
5 Breath control: 10 minutes
6 Full relaxation: 10 minutes

Preparation and positions

Long before you can attempt meditation or visualization you must master the important stretches that are a preparation for working on the asanas, or yogic postures.

Preparation is an important part of yoga practice. The aim is to ensure that the body is flexible, and therefore not at risk of injury, and that the mind is free and receptive. Simple stretching is an excellent way to warm up before working through the asanas, so each yoga session begins with gentle stretching exercises.

You can try these exercises at home. All you need is a mat long enough to lie on, and a quiet, warm space where you will not be disturbed. Make sure that all electronic gadgets, including cell phones and computers, are turned off. Wear comfortable, loose clothing but leave your feet bare. Take a moment of quiet before you begin.

The first sequence begins with simple stretches, including the Gentle Twist. It leads up to the Tree, a yoga posture that trains the all-important sense of balance. The second exercise is the Cat, a simple exercise that stretches the spine and helps it to become less rigid. The breathing is important because, in addition to aiding concentration and relaxation, it teaches control of the abdominal muscles.

FIRST SEQUENCE

1 Stand tall with feet apart, weight evenly distributed between both feet.

2 Breathing in, raise both arms steadily, pressing your weight into your heels. Lower your arms, breathing out. Repeat three times.

3 (the Gentle Twist) Stand tall. As you breathe in, raise your left arm to shoulder level in front of you. Watch your hand as you turn slowly to the left while breathing out. Keep the shoulder relaxed and twist only as far as is comfortable. Breathe in as you return, then repeat on the right side. Repeat the whole exercise three times.

4 Move the feet farther apart. Breathe in while you raise the right arm and stretch the right side of the body from foot to fingertip. Lower the arm, breathing out. Repeat three times each side.

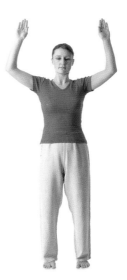

Most yoga sequences begin with simple stretching exercises.

5 (the Tree) Stand tall. Transfer your weight onto the right foot. Place the sole of your left foot on the inside of your right ankle, big toe just touching the ground, and turn the left knee out. Fix your gaze ahead and place your hands together at heart level. Hold this posture for three long breaths, then repeat on the other side.

THE CAT

1 Kneel with legs shoulder-width apart. Breathe out, placing your hands on the mat in line with the shoulders. Breathe in, lowering the back and raising the head. Hold this position.

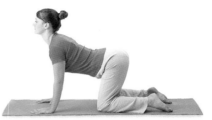

2 Breathe out while arching the back as high as possible and dropping your head between your arms. Hold this position and your breath for a few seconds. Repeat steps 1 and 2 between 10 and 20 times.

3 Sit back on the heels while moving your arms back. Rest the hands, palms up, beside heels. Lower your head until your forehead touches the mat. Before you get up relax, breathing gently, for a few moments.

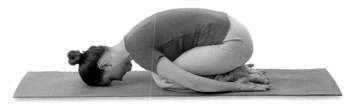

The Cat posture helps to restore the flexibility to a rigid spine.

Salute to the Sun

Yogis have found the Salute to the Sun extremely beneficial. Its roots are in sun worship and it is traditionally performed at dawn as a preparation for the asanas. In more recent times it has proved to be an excellent way to start the modern day.

The sequence of 12 stretches known as the Suryanamasakar, or Salute to the Sun, tones the muscles and improves respiration and heart rate. Experienced yogis can perform it as it is meant to be performed—rapidly and rhythmically—but the beginner should practice each movement separately, starting with the easiest ones.

Once you are familiar with the individual movements, try putting them together. At first, the full sequence may take several minutes to complete, but practice will improve fluidity and speed. The ultimate aim is to complete the full sequence in 20 seconds, but the Salute to the Sun demands great concentration to get the breathing right, so do not rush the process. The main purpose of the sequence is to energize.

SALUTE TO THE SUN

1 Stand tall but relaxed with your arms in Namaste, the prayer position. Breathe out.

2 Breathe in, raising your arms above your head. Link thumbs to stretch the spine. Keeping knees straight, lift the whole body.

3 Breathe out while swinging your body forward and down, head toward knees. Keep your legs straight, if possible, and place your hands on the floor beside your feet.

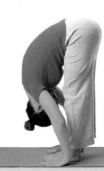

The Salute to the Sun is an invigorating way to get the day off to a good start.

The sequence stretches all the muscles in turn, beginning with the back muscles.

4 In a single movement, while breathing in, step forward, raising your trunk; bend your right knee, placing hands flat on the floor either side of the right foot, and stretch your left leg behind you. Weight is on the left foot and right hand, and the right knee is over the foot. Raise your head.

5 Pause, holding the breath and stretching your body. Move your right leg back in line with the left and raise your hips and legs from floor. Straighten the elbows and keep your head up.

6 Breathing out, descend to floor, knees first, then chest, then forehead. (The stomach does not touch the floor.)

7 Breathe in, stretching your feet back, raising your trunk and shoulders from floor.

8 Breathe in while sliding the toes forward until the balls of your feet are on the ground. Raise your hips, pushing your heels to the ground. Straighten your knees, contract stomach muscles, tuck your head between your arms. Hold the breath while stretching your whole body.

9 Breathe in, to perform position 4 but on the left-hand side.

10 Breathe out, bringing your right foot beside the left foot, hands flat on the floor, hips raised, knees straight, head tucked between your arms.

11 Breathe in deeply as you raise your trunk, hips, and arms and stretch forward and up. Link thumbs above your head, bending the spine back (as in step 2).

12 End the sequence by breathing out to stand erect with arms and hand in the prayer position.

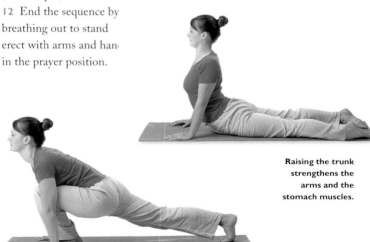

Raising the trunk strengthens the arms and the stomach muscles.

Steps 4 and 7 of the sequence stretch the thigh muscles and mobilize the hips.

Relaxation

Body and mind need to relax between asanas, and all yoga sessions are interspersed with periods of rest.

THE CORPSE

1 Sit on the floor, knees bent, feet flat on floor. Lean back, resting on your forearms.

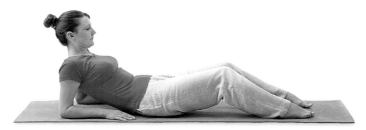

2 Move the forearms forward to allow the body to descend gently to the floor. Press back against the floor, then slide your feet forward. Press the backs of your knees against the floor, move your legs and arms out, and turn outward. Hands are palm up, with thumb and forefinger touching.

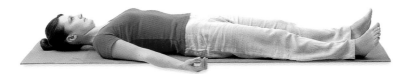

3 Close your eyes. Breathe gently and shallowly. Beginning with the toes, relax each part of your body in turn. It helps to tense the muscles and then relax them. Relax for 5–15 minutes, then stand slowly.

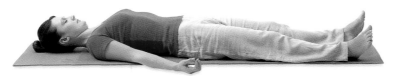

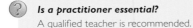

(?) **Is yoga is compatible with conventional medicine?**
Yes.

(?) **Is a practitioner essential?**
A qualified teacher is recommended.

ARTS
THERAPIES

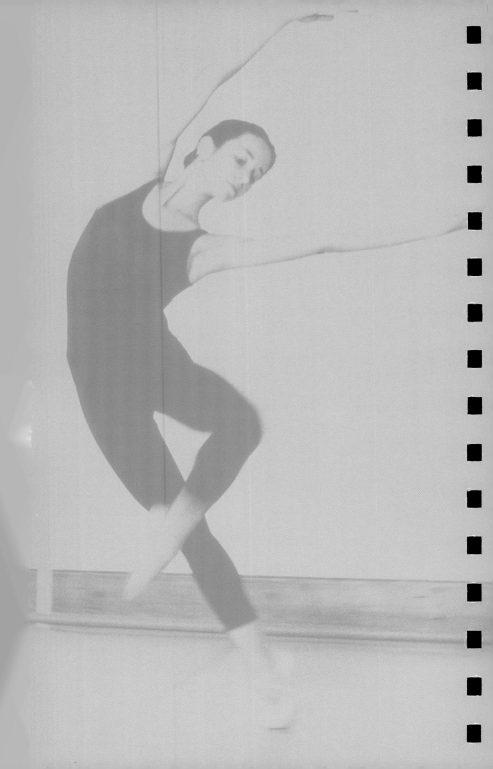

Not all therapies involve exercises or medication. Art, music, dance, and color therapies all tap into the creative wellspring at the heart of each human being, opening the door for creativity to express emotions or resolve conflicts that may be impossible to articulate in any other way. These therapies are particularly suitable for children, but can be used by anybody. Skill at art, music, or dance is unnecessary; the idea is to release the creative side of the mind in a therapeutic way. After a course, a person may never paint or dance or play an instrument again. Color therapy accesses the creative side in a rather indirect way, using light and color to calm, stimulate, or focus as necessary. For each of these therapies, a practitioner is essential to facilitate expression, provide suitable tools and techniques, and guide the session.

Dance movement therapy

In early times dance formed part of traditional healing practices and in some parts of the world these persist today in shamanistic rituals. The modern profession of dance movement therapy was born in the 1950s as a result of a union between dance and psychotherapy. While it bears many of the characteristics of these parents it has its own unique personality. Dance movement therapy is based on the holistic premise that posture and movement are indicative of, and influence, a person's mood and psychological functioning. In this form of therapy movement is a medium for self-expression, communication, and therapeutic intervention in the service of personal growth, integration, and healing.

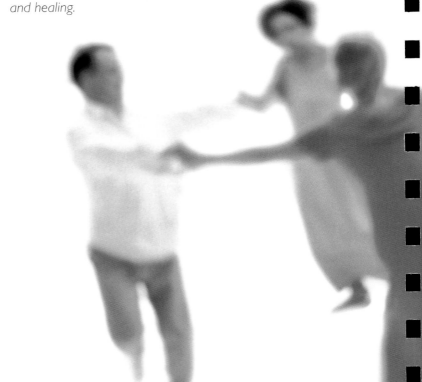

WILL IT HELP?

• Dance movement therapy provides a means of self-exploration and growth, leading to greater self-awareness and self-confidence.
• It can help to reestablish contact with sources of creativity and intuition and act as an antidote to stress.
• It is valuable in work with children.
• It is increasingly used as part of a multidisciplinary approach to treating patients with severe mental health problems such as schizophrenia, depression, and eating disorders.
• Its application to conditions such as chronic fatigue syndrome and psychosomatic illness is also being explored.

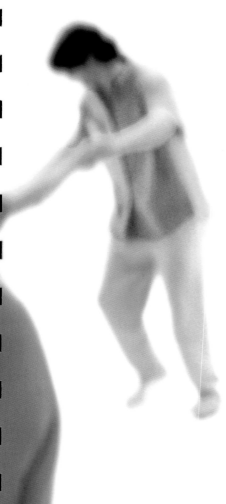

 BENEFITS

• The therapy can be practiced in both group and individual formats.
• Its nonverbal dimension can provide new insights about relationships with partners, friends, and business associates and can support the development of more adaptive ways of relating.

 CAUTION

• Check a therapist's qualifications before entering therapy. All dance movement therapists in private practice should have completed a postgraduate-level professional training of at least two years and be registered practitioner members of a professional association. Membership Registers are published by the American Dance Therapy Association.

Dance can bring the added benefit of social contact when performed as a group activity.

Most individual and group sessions comprise warm-up, process, and verbal phases.

• During warm-up the therapist may provide suggestions to help you warm up your body and make a transition into the process stage.
• During process you are invited to move in a spontaneous way, allowing movement to arise in response to bodily sensation, from an image, or in response to other group members. This stage has been compared to free association in verbal therapies. The therapist may intervene either verbally or through movement in response to your movement patterns, for example, to suggest you explore a movement pattern or theme.
• Toward the end of the session you are encouraged to reflect verbally on your experience and its significance for you, making links between patterns emerging in the sessions and those in your life outside therapy.

Movement and emotion

Dance movement therapy is a form of therapy that may be used to bring about change in emotional and psychological functioning through the use of expressive movement within the context of a therapeutic relationship. It draws on three main fields of practice, those of movement observation, psychology, and dance.

Posture and bodily movement are sensitive, unique indicators of personal style. The way we move tells those around us, usually at a subconscious level, the kind of person we are and something of our mood. In our encounters with others we both observe and sense such factors as the degree of focus in our own movement, the forcefulness or sensitivity, the sense of urgency or indulgence, the tightness or easy-going flow. We use this encoded information in forming our first impressions of people. The dance movement therapist's skills in movement observation and analysis enable a more differentiated awareness of such information to form the basis of an initial assessment and of subsequent interventions designed to help clients develop insight into their ways of moving through life.

DEVELOPMENT THERAPY Our experience of our own bodies forms the basis of our sense of identity. Body movement is our first language, mediating our first relationships and laying the foundations for our emotional, social, and cognitive development. The dance movement therapist works with an understanding of these developmental aspects of movement, particularly when working with children. The creative and playful use of movement can enable children to share their inner world with the therapist, who can then guide further therapeutic interventions. The therapist's skills in building relationships in this way have been found valuable in work with autistic and other nonverbal children. The playful and creative aspects of the therapy make it attractive for children with learning difficulties or emotional and behavioral disorders.

Therapeutic relationship

Dance movement therapists may draw on one of the psychological models of therapy, such as psychoanalytic, Jungian, or gestalt, to guide an understanding of the client and the process of therapy. Directness and immediacy in dance movement therapy characterize its nature. All approaches place importance on regular meetings at a set time and place, and a confidential relationship.

Dance movement therapists do not teach dance; rather, the client's own freely improvised body movement is used as a starting point for exploration of personal themes through movement, or for the exploration of relationships with others. There is a close connection between movement and feelings that facilitates the integration of feelings and insight so vital to therapeutic change. In this way dance movement therapy is helpful for clients who feel disconnected from their bodies and feelings.

 Is dance movement therapy compatible with conventional medicine?
Yes. Dance movement therapy addresses the whole person, influencing their mood and outlook, and encouraging the healing process.

 Is a practitioner necessary?
Yes. Participation in any form of dance brings feelings of well-being and improved self-esteem; likewise, engaging in creative activity can also have therapeutic benefits. It is the harnessing of the many aspects of dance and the creative process under the guidance of a trained therapist, however, that distinguishes dance movement therapy.

Color therapy

Light is a powerful form of energy that pervades our lives day after day. It is abundant, available, and absolutely free. Although its healing properties have been used, by a very few, for hundreds of years it is a medicine not of the past but of the future, and its therapeutic value is only now being realized.

Light sustains life on this planet, and is needed by almost all living things. The sun and its radiating energy are accepted as life's ordering force. Researchers have undertaken investigations into the healing properties of sunlight, but so far little study has been carried out into the value of its component colors. As minds open, so will the possibilities of using this gift of nature as a therapy that is easily accessible, gentle, and safe.

The sun's light takes eight and a half minutes to travel the 93,000,000 miles (150 million km) to earth, and without this energy nothing would survive. Our eyes filter this light to produce the visible colors of the spectrum.

Color therapy in nature: the stunning hues of sunset provide an inspiring display that lifts the emotions. Color therapists believe that color has an effect on mind, body, and spirit, and use it to restore health.

WILL IT HELP?

- Color therapy, like all holistic medicines, does not work on the body's physiology in isolation, but also causes a reaction on the emotional and psychological systems.
- This form of therapy is of immense value in redressing the balance of the mind, body, and soul.
- Each different color has a specific effect on each system, and within every color there are hundreds of tints and shades, which can have incredible healing properties with vast possibilities.

BENEFITS

- Color helps to balance a system that is in trauma. By working holistically color therapy can work through one system and affect another.
- It is used locally or systemically, or both, with good results.

CAUTION

- Because the potencies within each color cause an effect on every system, color therapy should be used with care and respect. There are side effects to all powerful medicines, however gentle.

Healing light

The healing properties of sunlight have been used for centuries. The sun was revered by early civilizations as the source of life, and understandably so. Light hits our planet at 186,000 miles (300,000 km) a second, having left the sun as radiation, 93 million miles (150 million km) away. This incredible electromagnetic energy reaches the Earth in eight and a half minutes, where it sustains all manner of life.

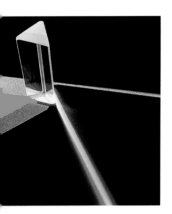

White light, passed through a prism, divides into seven spectral colors.

THE COLORS OF LIGHT In the 17th century Isaac Newton discovered the different frequencies within white light, the rainbow colors that appear in the sequence of red, orange, yellow, green, blue, indigo, and violet. Some spectral scales include blue-green and yellow-green. These are the colors used by color therapists, who often also add magenta—a synthesized color not found naturally in the visible spectrum. The palette of light that most color therapists use also includes turquoise, lemon, pink, and other colors created from the seven basic spectral colors. Color therapists believe that each has a healing value and is a crucial fuel for the maintenance of health.

Medical use of light

Blue light is commonly used to treat neonatal jaundice. More than 60 percent of premature babies suffer from this condition, caused by the buildup of a yellow body chemical, bilirubin. Blue light, shone over the body, breaks down the bilirubin, enabling the baby to eliminate it safely.

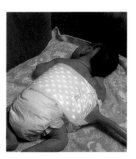

Babies born with jaundice are healed with blue light.

Leg ulcers may be treated with red light, which increases the local blood supply, cleaning and healing the affected area. Red flickering light is used for premenstrual syndrome, and a steady red frequency can ease pain from serious burns. Mainstream medicine often uses ultraviolet (UV) light for acne and psoriasis, and low-level (soft) laser encourages deep bruise and wound healing.

Color therapy treatments

Different colors stimulate the nervous system and can raise or lower blood pressure and respiratory and pulse rates. Yellow, orange, and red stimulate, and green and blue are physiological calmatives, corresponding to the emotional effects they have long been known to have.

Light can be given to the patient through the eyes, and many color therapists use this treatment method. Not all light entering the eyes is for seeing: 20 percent passes through the back of the retina and onto the hypothalamus in the brain.

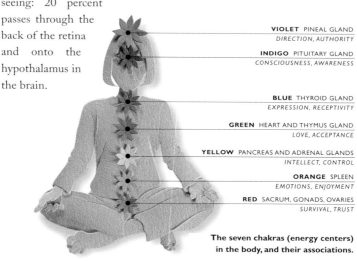

VIOLET PINEAL GLAND
DIRECTION, AUTHORITY

INDIGO PITUITARY GLAND
CONSCIOUSNESS, AWARENESS

BLUE THYROID GLAND
EXPRESSION, RECEPTIVITY

GREEN HEART AND THYMUS GLAND
LOVE, ACCEPTANCE

YELLOW PANCREAS AND ADRENAL GLANDS
INTELLECT, CONTROL

ORANGE SPLEEN
EMOTIONS, ENJOYMENT

RED SACRUM, GONADS, OVARIES
SURVIVAL, TRUST

**The seven chakras (energy centers)
in the body, and their associations.**

The hypothalamus is involved in the regulation of the automatic nervous system, body temperature, appetite, thirst, blood flow, emotions, and sex drive, and in the control of the pituitary gland. Color therapists believe that light energy somehow stimulates the glands into functioning properly, thus regulating balance.

Some color therapists irradiate light directly through the patient's skin, covering the eyes completely. Others work with a system of chakras. These are believed to be entry points into the body through which light can be absorbed and channeled via a network of meridians that pervade the body, to reach and heal any imbalances. Another method of treatment is through an energy field, or aura, believed to surround every human being. Our state of health is reflected as different colors, visible to certain gifted people, within this surrounding field. A therapist might pass color through, or into, the patient's aura to redress an imbalance in the system; while a small area in need of treatment may be given local irradiation.

COLOR DIAGNOSIS

When treating emotional or psychological imbalance the therapist might work through chakras, aura, or the physical body, depending on the diagnosis. Color has long been known to have the potential to affect our moods, feelings and general state of mind—even our conscious choices, as any advertising company knows. Important work carried out by leading psychologists into these effects has led to the development of some color psychology tests, and these are used as a diagnostic tool by a number of color therapists. The method of diagnosing for a color patient depends largely on the practitioner. Some dowse with a pendulum, others look at the patient's aura. A few prefer to work with a medical diagnosis.

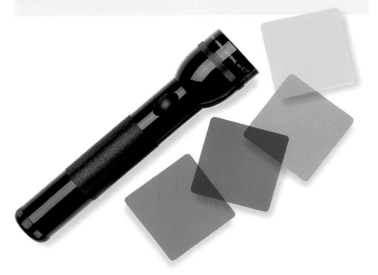

A flashlight and some colored filters are all you need to make up a color therapy kit for use at home.

Equipment for treatment

The equipment of a color therapist or light therapist ranges from large electric lamps, down to tiny torches, but each type of light/color source uses colored filters or lenses to obtain the exact color needed for the patient. Different imbalances require different equipment. In the treatment of seasonal affective disorder (SAD), for instance, very powerful doses of full spectrum light (white) are given to suppress the secretions of melatonin, a hormone released by the pineal gland in the brain that causes drowsiness. On the other hand, treating a baby might require very small doses of unsaturated (pale) colors.

Therapy and self-help

There are several recognized professional bodies of color/light therapists in existence. Before visiting a therapist it is worth checking whether he or she is a member of one of these recognized bodies.

As an alternative to visiting a trained color therapist, it is possible to gain enough knowledge through studying some of the informative books that are available to treat yourself for many imbalances. The only equipment needed is a light source, such as a table lamp or flashlight, and a selection of colored filters, such as those used for stage lighting. As with all complementary medicine, it is wise also to consult a conventional medical practitioner for any serious health problem.

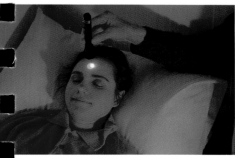

In a magenta room, yellow light is directed at the brow chakra.

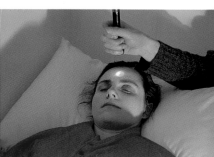

Chakras are believed to channel light to where it is needed for healing.

A colorful future

Nobody really knows exactly how color medicine works, and more research is needed into this marvelous therapy. The most effective color therapy developed to date is the Spectro-Chrome system of the pioneer Dinshah Ghadiali. He hoped to see this therapy used in every home, and left important knowledge to those who seek an enlightened path in the art of healing. Light gives life itself: what better medicine could there be?

Is color therapy compatible with conventional medicine?
Color therapy is a type of energy medicine, and will not interfere with any conventional medical treatment.

Is a practitioner necessary?
A practitioner is recommended but not essential.

Art therapy

Art therapy is based on the belief that psychic experience can be reached and expressed through images, whether they be the scribbles of a toddler or the work of a sculptor. As the psychoanalyst listens to the dream, so the art therapist looks at the image, and together therapist and client begin to understand the inner world of the client. While ten people might describe themselves as "depressed," they will each make a different image of their depression. Fortunately being "good at art" is absolutely unnecessary—anyone who can pick up a pencil or make a mark in clay can participate.

What is art therapy?

Art therapy has its roots in various disciplines including psychoanalysis, psychiatry, and art teaching. Used originally as a diagnostic tool in psychiatric hospitals, it has, during recent years, gained recognition as a treatment in its own right.

Underlying current practice are a number of key principles. There is general acceptance that it is the therapeutic rather than the aesthetic value of the art produced that is important. This is important since it means that artistic ability bears no relation to the capacity to benefit from art therapy.

Fundamental to art therapy is the belief that the capacity to make marks is virtually universal, and that such mark-making can develop into a symbolic language, capable of being understood. Art therapy believes that there are aspects of ourselves that are beyond our conscious awareness, and that these can be accessed via symbols that are thrown up by the unconscious. In art therapy the vehicle for such symbolic expression is the image made by the client.

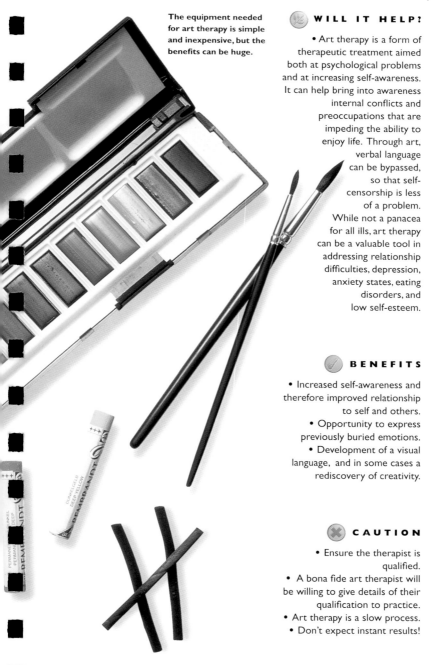

The equipment needed for art therapy is simple and inexpensive, but the benefits can be huge.

WILL IT HELP?

• Art therapy is a form of therapeutic treatment aimed both at psychological problems and at increasing self-awareness. It can help bring into awareness internal conflicts and preoccupations that are impeding the ability to enjoy life. Through art, verbal language can be bypassed, so that self-censorship is less of a problem. While not a panacea for all ills, art therapy can be a valuable tool in addressing relationship difficulties, depression, anxiety states, eating disorders, and low self-esteem.

BENEFITS

• Increased self-awareness and therefore improved relationship to self and others.
• Opportunity to express previously buried emotions.
• Development of a visual language, and in some cases a rediscovery of creativity.

CAUTION

• Ensure the therapist is qualified.
• A bona fide art therapist will be willing to give details of their qualification to practice.
• Art therapy is a slow process.
• Don't expect instant results!

Media

Any media can be used for the expression of feeling. Most commonly available are paints, pencil, charcoal, paper, cardboard and clay. In some settings a far broader range of media are available, permitting work that is experimental in the broadest sense. There might be the opportunity to work on a huge scale, or to create using material not usually associated with conventional art classes. Either way, it is not an impressive array of art materials that matters, but the experience of creating in the context of a safe, therapeutic relationship, with a practitioner who can, over time, develop an understanding of each individual's visual language; the recurring themes that emerge and their symbolic significance.

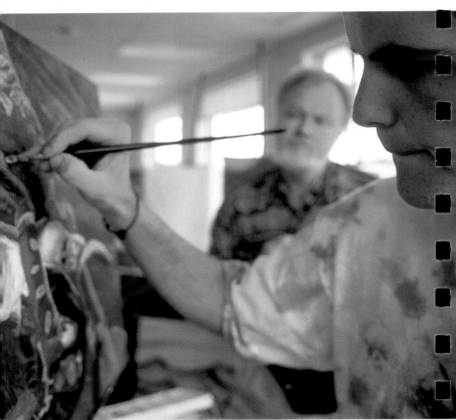

In art therapy, it is the therapeutic
value of expression that is important,
not the artistic skill.

The relationship with the therapist is central to progress. It is the therapist who creates the setting, both physically and psychologically, in which the client may, over time, feel safe enough to express powerful emotions. Through the holding capacity of that relationship and the images themselves, there is the opportunity to express feelings that might ordinarily be felt to be too threatening, whether they are positive or negative. Feelings of love and hate, desire and aggression, anger, fear, and grief can be contained in the art therapy setting.

Art therapy in action

Art therapy has many different applications and is used with a wide range of client groups. These include those suffering serious mental illnesses, men and women in prison, adults and children with learning difficulties, the elderly, the speech impaired, and the dying. It is, however, increasingly used with individuals who seek to increase their own level of self-awareness and want to address the difficulties in their lives in a creative way.

Art therapy is conducted both in groups and one-to-one settings, and each has its own advantages. In the group situation the dynamics of the group itself become part of the therapeutic work and the individual learns about how he or she functions in a group setting. There is less individual attention but a greater sense of not being alone. There is a chance both to give and to receive. In individual therapy there is total privacy and exclusive individual attention, with no need to wait for or share the attention of the therapist. Group sessions are generally longer than individual.

There are different schools and styles of art therapy, some humanistic and some psychoanalytic. Some therapists are directive and structure the session for the client, others work nondirectly and work with whatever comes up. Another difference concerns the extent to which the therapist considers the therapeutic relationship to be important over and above the art image. What is common among the therapists is the use of the art image as a means of communication in addition to words.

Is art therapy compatible with conventional medicine?
Art therapy addresses the overall emotional needs of the patient rather than specific conditions, so that it complements conventional treatment.

Is a practitioner necessary?
Yes, the relationship between therapist and patient is crucial to progress.

Music therapy

The link between music and healing has been recognized for thousands of years and throughout all societies. The sounds which constitute music—rhythm, pitch, harmony, and timbre—resonate with the rhythms and sonorities of the human body. This is experienced by people of all ages, from the fetus in the womb to the person approaching the end of life. Evidence has shown that the ability to respond to music is not impaired by illness, trauma, or disability, so that music therapy is an effective form of treatment for people with a wide range of needs and conditions. Music therapy has its roots in ancient times but over the last 50 years has developed professional training courses, a career structure, and research which has confirmed its effectiveness.

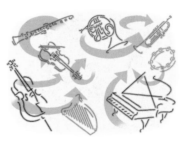

The cadences of music help restore rhythm to life by putting you in tune with the vibrations of the body.

Overview of music therapy

The key principle of music therapy is the use of music and sounds within a relationship between therapist and client to support and encourage physical, psychological, social, and emotional well-being. Music used in the clinical setting engages clients and enables changes to take place which may be on a physical or psychological level.

Music therapy takes place on a one-to-one basis or in a small group. Patients can be referred via their own physician, a psychiatrist, a pediatrician, or a hospital consultant. In the Education Service music therapists work mainly in special schools and nurseries, though there are some within special units of mainstream schools, for children with, for example, language disorders, sensory impairment, or behavior problems. Social services also refer clients for music therapy, as does the prison service.

WILL IT HELP?

• Music therapists are usually trained musicians who have completed a postgraduate training course to equip them to offer music therapy to children and adults of all ages. They work with people with a wide range of difficulties including learning disability, autism, developmental delay, communication disorders, depression, mental health problems, dementia, and terminal illness. Other categories include people with eating disorders, children who have suffered neglect or abuse, juvenile delinquents and prisoners, and patients in nursing homes.

 BENEFITS

• While music therapy may relieve specific symptoms, for example, by relaxing physical tension or alleviating anxiety, the therapist is generally working with the whole person, addressing needs which are personal to the individual client. The gains and benefits of music therapy will not be of a specifically musical nature but may be experienced in any of the following areas: Communication • A sense of self • Self-expression • Relationships • Creativity • Self-confidence

CAUTION

• When looking for a music therapist, always contact a registered and qualified practitioner.

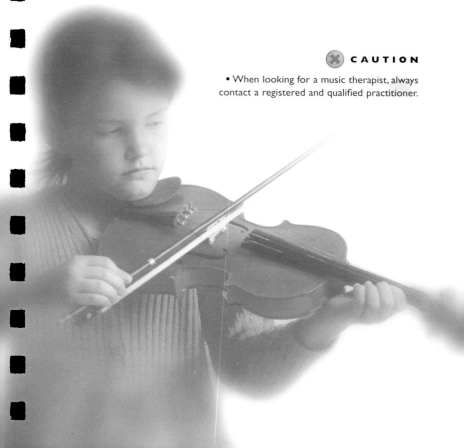

It is not necessary to be musical to take part in a music therapy session. The therapist will use his or her own instrument and will invite the client to join in the improvised music using accessible instruments, such as percussion and ethnic instruments. The therapist and client may also sing or move with the music. Music is a nonverbal means of communication, but the client and therapist may talk during the session, or may remain silent.

After the initial referral, there will generally be a period of assessment, after which a contract will be drawn up for future sessions. As therapy is an on-going process, clients are encouraged to commit themselves to a period of regular therapy which may last weeks, months, or years, depending on the nature of the problem.

Different approaches

Music is a very flexible medium and the practitioner will adapt his or her approach according to the needs of the client group. For example, a group of preschool children with developmental delay would need a different experience from an adolescent with anorexia or an elderly person with Alzheimer's disease. With young children the element of "play" in music is very important; for older people reminiscence and memories of the past may be significant. For people with emotional or psychological illnesses, music therapy can be a safe place in which to explore their fears, anxiety, or anger.

Self-help or practitioner led?

Whether through listening to music, playing, singing, or dancing, most people have had the experience of music being therapeutic and beneficial. Where music therapy differs from this kind of self-help is that in a therapy session the therapist is present to establish an interaction and a shared creative experience with the client. The sessions also take place within an agreed therapeutic framework of regularity and consistency. In addition, part of the therapist's professional ethos will be to liaise with other members of the therapeutic, educational, or medical team where appropriate.

 Is music therapy compatible with conventional medicine?
Music therapy addresses the overall emotional needs of the patient rather than specific conditions, so that it complements conventional treatment.

 Is a practitioner necessary?
Yes, the therapist establishes a context for the patient's creativity.

MIND

THERAPIES

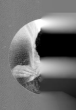

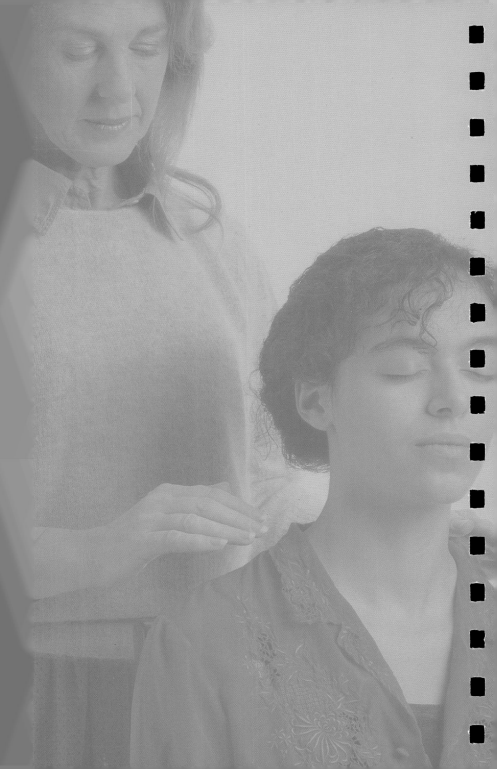

Some therapies are designed to work through the mind, rather than the body, to harness the power of the mind to influence action and development in the body. Psychotherapy and hypnotherapy are two well-known, established therapies accepted by mainstream medicine; healing requires more of a leap of faith and not everyone can make it. Psychotherapy in particular has now proliferated into many schools and approaches, while hypnotherapy is more straightforward. Healing, usually considered a gift or talent by a healer, is by its nature not open to much regulation. A practitioner is essential for all three therapies—although hypnotherapy can be self-applied after guidance—but since the nature of these techniques leaves them open to abuse by charlatans, a therapist's qualifications should be rigorously checked.

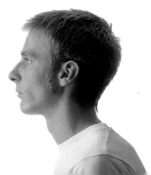

Healing

Traditional healing has been practiced for many thousands of years and its existence has been recorded in cultures and religions throughout the world. Nowadays it is practiced from a variety of traditions—from spiritual healing to reiki and therapeutic touch—and it is often present in other therapies, especially if rapport with the patient is important or where some form of touch is involved.

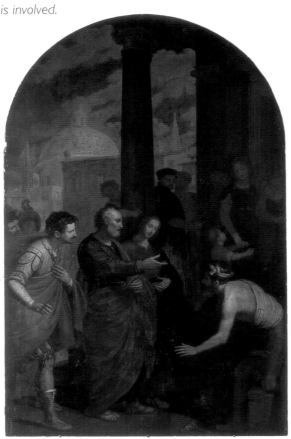

Healing has been traditionally associated with religious faith. The Bible, for example, contains many dramatic stories of healing.

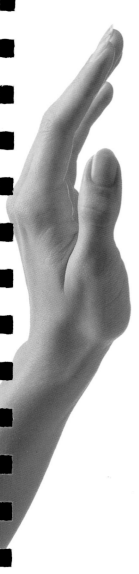

 ## WILL IT HELP?

- Healing is completely natural and noninvasive.
- It is a powerful relaxant and a powerful restorative.
- Healing aims to address the fundamental sources of ill health. It can therefore be helpful in a wide range of illnesses, both physical and psychological, sometimes to a remarkable degree.
- Healing complements both conventional medical treatment and other complementary therapies, or can be employed as a stand-alone treatment.

 ## BENEFITS

- Healing has no known undesirable side effects.
- Although a result is never guaranteed, recipients of healing rarely fail to benefit from it, for instance from an increased feeling of well-being and inner strength.

 ## CAUTION

- Healers complement the work of the medical profession and it is advisable to remain in touch with your doctor in case your illness calls for medical intervention.

Healing results from the interchange of energy between the healer and the recipient.

How healing works

The practice of healing seeks to trigger a natural process, to destress, to restore balance within the body (homeostasis), to restore the patient's ability to "self-heal," to help his or her immune system. In simple terms the body "knows" how to deal with a broken bone or a cut finger and it is this natural ability to "repair" ourselves that the healer seeks to stimulate.

The interaction between doctors and nurses and other carers and their patients often triggers a "healing" response and we all know that the proximity of friends and loved ones can have a healing effect. The qualities these situations seem to have in common are twofold, namely an active relationship and the presence of beneficial intent. Within traditional healing, the healer employs these in a deliberate way that enhances their therapeutic effect. He or she sets up an energetic interaction with the patient, reinforced by focussed intent.

The treatment

What happens during a session of healing? Firstly the healer may wish to understand your difficulty and explain what is going to happen, and will want to relax you. All that is required of the patient, however, is openness, a degree of confidence in the healer, and sometimes a willingness to change. Faith as such is not usually expected or necessary, but if the healer and patient happen to share a common religious belief, for example, this can be helpful in establishing a positive rapport

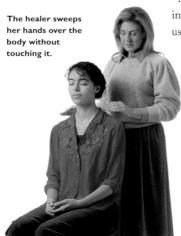

The healer sweeps her hands over the body without touching it.

Although healing can be practiced informally under any conditions, it is usually carried out with the patient seated on a chair or lying on a treatment couch: there is no need to remove clothing, except perhaps for heavy outerwear. The treatment will begin with the healer relaxing and concentrating on the patient and then passing his or her hands at varying distances above the body. Sometimes light touch is also used. Sessions usually last from 20 minutes to half an hour, but can be shorter or longer according to the condition being treated and the judgement of the healer. The resulting interaction between healer and patient seems to restore and reinvigorate the patient, with the results that have been described.

Both healer and recipient can experience a variety of sensations while the treatment takes place, including tingling and pressure, changes of temperature, and subtle pulsations on the surface of the body. At the end of the session the patient usually feels profoundly relaxed and a feeling of being reenergized or renewed often follows on the morning after the session. But the course of a patient's condition following a session is virtually impossible to predict—effects have been noted immediately, overnight, days later, and even weeks later. It is rare for patients not to be affected in some beneficial way. Many healers work with focussed intent at a distance—known as distant healing. This too has proved remarkably effective. Sometimes several sessions are needed and this is something for discussion between healer and patient.

Healing sometimes results in an abreaction or a release of suppressed symptoms which is part of the patient's recovery process, making him or her feel worse before feeling better. It can also sometimes expose a condition which needs medical attention. So it is always advisable for patients to remain in touch with their doctor in case some form of medical intervention is indicated.

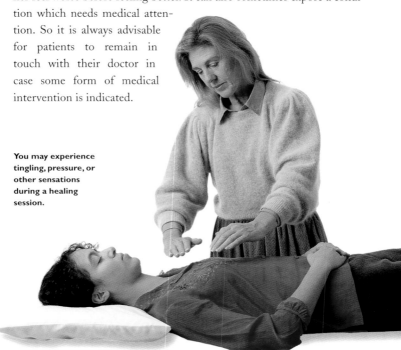

You may experience tingling, pressure, or other sensations during a healing session.

The scientific evidence

Healing has been proven scientifically to bring about a beneficial effect on stressed or damaged enzymes, seeds, yeasts, bacteria, plants, and animals, and to accelerate the healing of simple injuries in humans. Scientific evidence for the ability of directed intent—and especially prayer—to effect change is accumulating. In his comprehensive review of over 175 controlled studies of healing, Dr. Daniel Benor identified over half which demonstrated significant results.

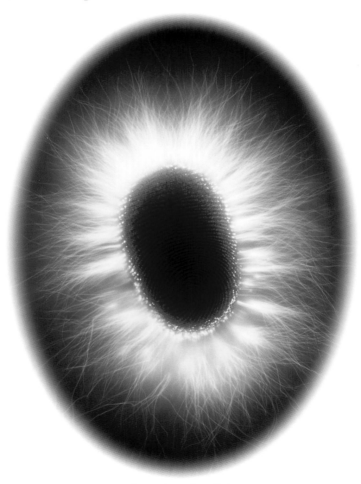

**Power at your fingertips?
This image of electromagnetic
discharge confirms it.**

Healing is a challenging area for scientific investigation. In medicine a specific treatment is prescribed to produce a specific outcome. Healing works differently. It seeks to trigger a spontaneous reaction in the body ,which helps the natural self-healing mechanism to address malfunction at all levels more effectively. As a consequence the patient experiences benefit in ways other than, or in addition to, any effect on the presenting symptom or injury itself. And the interaction between the healer and the patient is a unique one.

Interest in healing and the scientific evidence supporting its efficacy continues to grow. But leaving aside the question of scientific evidence, experience over many years bears witness to its effectiveness. The best evidence for the patient is often self-evidence: to experience it oneself.

Finding a healer

Healing is a natural ability and many more individuals can give healing than actually practice it. Many healers work informally. There is also a growing interest in practicing healing among doctors, nurses, physiotherapists, and other healthcare professionals. An increasing number of family doctors include healers in their complementary therapy team and most nursing homes make healing available to their patients.

Healers belonging to organizations affiliated to the Confederation of Healing Organizations (CHO) have their skills properly validated, serve a two-year probationary period supervised by experienced colleagues, and undertake training courses to enhance their ability. Membership involves mandatory compliance with a Code of Conduct, and insurance to practice. Many healers are also trained in counseling.

Selection of a healer is always ultimately a matter for personal choice. Personal recommendation is often used, but lists of healers can be obtained from the healing organizations. Good healing can perhaps be best summed up in three words: energy, empathy, and understanding.

Is healing compatible with conventional medicine?
Healing complements conventional medical treatment, and your physician should be kept informed of any changes in a specific condition.

Is a practitioner necessary?
Yes. The healer acts to stimulate the patient's own self-healing energies, and part of this process is relational.

Psychotherapy

The psyche is closely associated with our sense of identity and meaning in life and its need for therapy comes from the fact that we can suffer inward pain, inner conflict, and feelings of alienation. Virtually all cultures have had methods of addressing the troubles of the soul or psyche, the most common being religious and mystical rituals; supporting relationships with family, friends, and mentors; and the

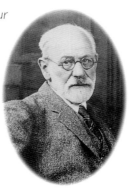

Sigmund Freud (1856–1939) was the founder of psychoanalysis.

use of mood-altering substances and medications. In modern Western society medications for psychological troubles are increasingly available but there has been a weakening of family networks and a decline in religion. Psychotherapy provides a supporting relationship and offers a

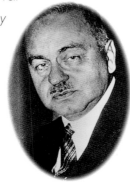

Carl Jung (1875–1961) developed the concepts of introvert and extrovert.

largely secular approach to the care of the soul and its troubles. During the twentieth century it has been formalized and developed into a number of distinctive methods, each based on a particular view of the human psyche.

Alfred Adler (1870–1939) came up with the theory of the inferiority complex.

WILL IT HELP?

• Psychotherapy can treat behavioral, emotional, and sexual disorders, personality disorders, nervous disorders (neuroses), problems of psychological development, and all other non-organic mental problems.
• Forms of psychotherapy can be helpful in times of crisis, such as during bereavement or severe illness.
• The goal of psychotherapy is to bring about clarity, inner harmony, and self-understanding in place of confusion, conflict, and alienation.
• The therapy works through the therapeutic alliance between the therapist and the client.
This mobilizes the client's thinking and emotional processes to create changes in understanding, feelings, and behavior.

Lurking fears may send you hurtling into a dark tunnel, but psychotherapy can show you the way out.

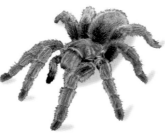

BENEFITS

• Clients are empowered and liberated from self-destructive beliefs and thinking patterns.
• Mental or emotional stress is alleviated.
• There may also be physical benefits, where there has been a psychosomatic element in a physical complaint.

CAUTION

• Choose the therapy and therapist with care. Bear in mind that there are many forms of psychotherapy available and aim to select one that matches both your needs and your financial resources.
• Problems with a major biological base (e.g. schizophrenia) will continue to require medication during psychotherapy.

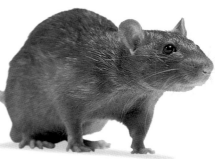

An interactive therapy

The beneficial effects of psychotherapy come about through a fruitful interaction between the therapist and the client. The therapist–client relationship may incorporate elements found in traditional social relationships, such as teacher–pupil, parent–child, partners-in-a-project, friend–friend, or confidant–confider.

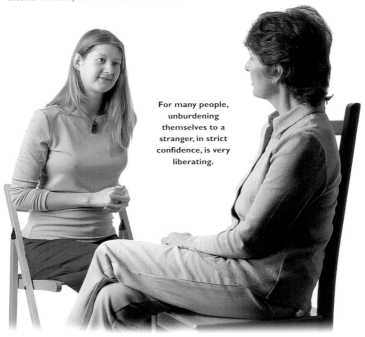

For many people, unburdening themselves to a stranger, in strict confidence, is very liberating.

The therapist–client relationship

Particular conditions apply to this specialized relationship, whatever its precise form. However, as well as one-to-one, therapeutic relations can include a group of clients with one or more therapists leading sessions; client families with one or more therapists, and intensive therapeutic relationships in residential settings. Most major forms of psychotherapy discourage any significant departures from the following boundaries:

• the therapist observes strict confidence

• there is a planned and structured interaction, aimed at promoting changes in the client's attitudes, beliefs, thinking, and behavior

• the interaction is confined to prearranged sessions of a fixed duration, in return for which the therapist receives payment.

Types of psychotherapy

Over 300 different types of psychotherapy are currently available, with major variations between them. Some of the most influential branches are briefly described here.

Behavioral psychology emphasizes the therapist's teaching role in designing and implementing a program by which the client "unlearns" undesirable behavior and "learns" desirable behavior. The focus is on the behavior itself rather than underlying causes. Undesirable behavior is discouraged through association with punishment or absence of reward, while desirable behavior is encouraged through reward. This may consist simply of the therapist's approval or attention, or may involve a program of agreed treats on goal achievement. Behavioral psychotherapy is used for clients with clearly defined problems for which a suitable programme can be designed, such as phobias, social skills deficits, habit disorders, eating disorders, and forms of sexual dysfunction or compulsive behavior. Behavioral psychotherapy is a relatively short-term treatment, often lasting only a few months.

In analytical psychotherapy the emphasis is on revealing the hidden causes of conflict within the client. This form of therapy seeks to achieve awareness of unconscious processes as a means of bringing about change. During sessions, the client is encouraged to recall dreams or produce seemingly "random" thoughts and memories, which are considered to come from the unconscious part of the mind and are interpreted by the analyst to reveal their inner meaning. Depending on the particular school of analysis, the emphasis may be on sexual dynamics within the family

Be very clear about what you are embarking on before you begin therapy. Make detailed enquiries about duration of treatment and cost, and the therapist's view of the relationship that will develop between you. Ask who will decide when the therapy should end, how progress will be monitored and who will decide whether it is satisfactory. Be sure that you will be happy working in the way proposed by the therapist.

Don't ignore your feelings if you are unhappy or uneasy about any aspect of your therapeutic relationship and cannot resolve this with your therapist. You are the customer, and you can take your custom elsewhere. At the same time, be aware that, to be productive, the therapeutic process will almost certainly involve working through some difficulties and that this may be painful at times.

USING PSYCHOTHERAPY

(Freud), competitive dynamics in relations with siblings and others (Adler), or movements within the self to correct imbalance and fulfill its potential (Jung). Therapy can last for a number of years and in many cases three or more sessions weekly are recommended.

Humanistic or integrative psychotherapy is based on a positive view of the potential of the human psyche for growth and "self-actualization." The process of working toward this is often described as "integration," with an assumption that no element of the psyche, however apparently undesirable, should be rejected and that such elements can be integrated into a harmonious whole through the resolution of inner conflicts. The therapeutic relationship is viewed as a partnership, with the therapist facilitating rather than directing the development of the client's own psychological processes. Overtly "spiritual" elements are more likely to be encountered in this approach. The therapy is flexible in length, with the "partner" relationship being open to client-initiated breaks and termination. It can last for a number of years, but there is much variety, and some methods offer short, intensive courses.

Cognitive psychotherapy emphasizes the effect of patterns of thinking on feeling and behavior. The assumption is that behind problematic feeling and behavior there is an irrational thinking pattern. Its aim is to lead the client to examine these underlying thoughts with a view to replacing them with a more constructive pattern. The therapist takes a role similar to that of a coach, aiming to direct the client toward exercising his or her own rational faculties and taking responsibility for his or her actions. Therapy is goal-directed and change-oriented, with minimal dwelling on the client's past history, and is often of relatively short duration.

Counseling shares many elements with psychotherapy, especially the development of a supportive relationship between counselor and client. Counseling tends to be a more general form of helping that can be adapted to many specialized situations where psychological distress is encountered, such as in debt counseling or work-related counseling. Counselors vary in orientation along similar lines to psychotherapists, but a very influential approach is that developed by Carl Rogers, who believed that clients need unconditional acceptance and positive regard from the therapist/counselor. Counselors following his approach often reflect back the client's own statements to facilitate greater self-awareness, with the aim of encouraging the client to accept himself or herself to reduce inner conflict. Counseling is available for variable durations, from short fixed-term contracts to a number of years.

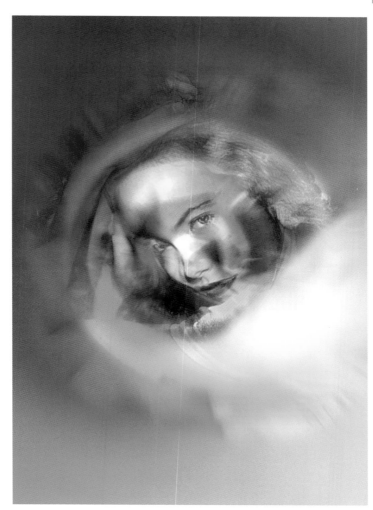

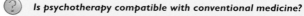

? *Is psychotherapy compatible with conventional medicine?*
Psychotherapy focuses on mental and emotional rather than physiological
problems; some conditions may also require medical treatment.

? *Is a practitioner necessary?*
Yes, all forms of psychotherapy work primarily through the relationship
between therapist and client.

Hypnotherapy

Hypnotherapy is the name given to the modern practice of hypnosis for therapeutic purposes. Hypnosis enables the everyday activity of the conscious mind to be reduced, giving the subject far greater access to the nonconscious parts of the mind. Under hypnosis (in trance), a person is more open emotionally, and more susceptible to suggestion, than in the normal waking state, and is generally more physically relaxed. Similar states, usually to a lighter degree, can occur spontaneously in everyday life, for instance, when daydreaming. This is a very favorable condition for gaining access to traumatic material and negative beliefs, for facilitating therapeutic reevaluation and reintegration of past experiences, and for helping to frame new attitudes, thinking, and behavior, and can be utilized and developed for many therapeutic purposes.

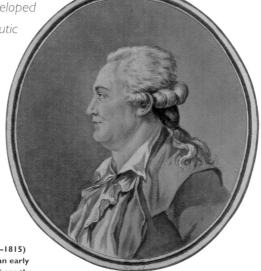

The Austrian physician Friedrich Mesmer (1734–1815) developed mesmerism, an early form of hypnotherapy where the therapist imposed his will on that of the patient through a hypnotic state.

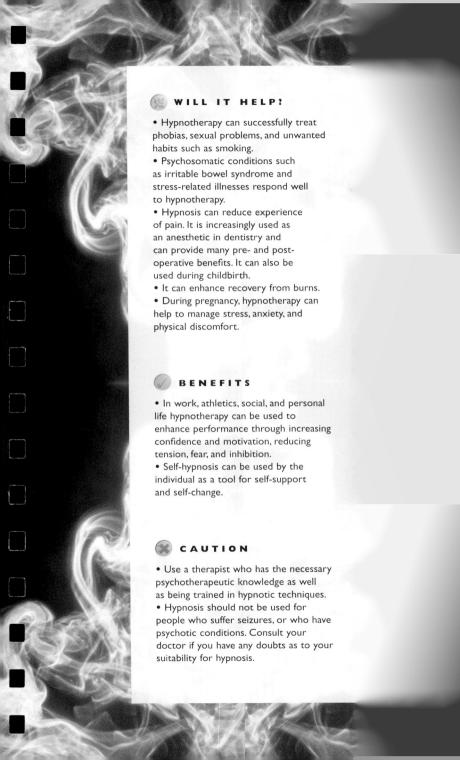

WILL IT HELP?

• Hypnotherapy can successfully treat phobias, sexual problems, and unwanted habits such as smoking.
• Psychosomatic conditions such as irritable bowel syndrome and stress-related illnesses respond well to hypnotherapy.
• Hypnosis can reduce experience of pain. It is increasingly used as an anesthetic in dentistry and can provide many pre- and post-operative benefits. It can also be used during childbirth.
• It can enhance recovery from burns.
• During pregnancy, hypnotherapy can help to manage stress, anxiety, and physical discomfort.

BENEFITS

• In work, athletics, social, and personal life hypnotherapy can be used to enhance performance through increasing confidence and motivation, reducing tension, fear, and inhibition.
• Self-hypnosis can be used by the individual as a tool for self-support and self-change.

CAUTION

• Use a therapist who has the necessary psychotherapeutic knowledge as well as being trained in hypnotic techniques.
• Hypnosis should not be used for people who suffer seizures, or who have psychotic conditions. Consult your doctor if you have any doubts as to your suitability for hypnosis.

Classic hypnotherapy

Classic hypnotherapy is one of the shorter psychological therapies, usually achieving its effects in one to eight sessions. The client achieves deeper hypnosis with repeated sessions, and between sessions the effects are reinforced by self-hypnosis, and perhaps an audio cassette recording of a session to listen to at home. Sessions are usually one-to-one but group sessions are sometimes given for aims such as giving up smoking, or problems such as irritable bowel syndrome. Techniques such as gestalt or analytic can also be used in hypnosis.

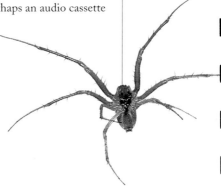

Sufferers of arachnophobia (fear of spiders) may respond to a course of hypnotherapy.

Therapy can take longer in the case of complex problems, or if apparently simple cases prove to be complicated by disturbing memories or negative feelings coming to light during or after hypnosis. This occurs in only a minority of cases and indicates that there are more complex issues involved, which need to be dealt with in order to achieve the therapeutic goals. In such cases regression in hypnosis may be used to facilitate recall of disturbing past events and help the client to gain an understanding of their effects on the present and make changes through the interpretation of these events. This approach is sometimes called hypnopsychotherapy.

Because of the possibility of psychological complications arising, it is advisable to seek hypnotherapy from a practitioner who can provide the appropriate psychological therapy. In all cases, a detailed consultation should be held at the outset, and monitoring should continue throughout.

CLIENT INVOLVEMENT

Hypnotherapy is an active process for the client; it is more helpful to look on it as a skill that you are going to learn with the aid of a coach and teacher rather than as something that is done to you. Practice between sessions and you will speed up your progress and strengthen your skills. Self-hypnosis gives you a valuable tool for life.

Hypnotherapy treatment

After the initial consultation, each therapeutic session consists of a number of different stages.

• The first is induction of hypnosis, most commonly by a verbal relaxation script designed to engage the attention of the client, but also sometimes by confusional techniques, "fixed gaze" or various rapid induction methods, although these are less commonly used by most therapists.

• Once the patient is under hypnosis, suggestions, and in more complex cases other therapeutic strategies also, are given in accordance with the client's therapeutic goals, e.g. to stop smoking or to gain confidence.

• The hypnosis is terminated by a process reversing the original induction, bringing the client back to full awareness, coupled with suggestions for feelings of well-being.

Post-hypnotic suggestions are given at the end of the session. For example, the client is reminded in the conscious state of suggestions given during hypnosis together with a suggestion that they will have effect after the hypnosis is terminated. Self-hypnosis can be taught by this method, with the client being given suggestions that he or she will be able to induce hypnosis in himself or herself and use it for relaxation and other therapeutic purposes.

The effectiveness of the therapy will depend on the responsiveness and commitment of the client, the degree of rapport between client and practitioner, and the skill and ability of the practitioner to perform the induction and provide therapeutic intervention, strategies, and suggestions in a way that is appropriate to the client.

SOME MISCONCEPTIONS

• Many people fear that they will "lose control" during hypnosis, but its effects are brought about by the cooperation of the client's own mind, and particularly his or her imagination. A properly trained practitioner makes it clear at all times that the client has the choice of whether to cooperate with suggestions made.

• It is a common misconception that through hypnosis a completely accurate memory recall may be obtained. In fact, while memory recall may be facilitated by hypnosis, imagination and fantasy can also be enhanced, resulting in confabulation. This may be very convincing but it is not factually accurate. No reputable hypnotherapist would claim to be able to retrieve an accurate memory picture through hypnosis.

Variations in practice

In the 1950s both the British Medical Association and the American Medical Association recommended hypnotherapy as a form of treatment, and today it is offered in many hospitals to help address a wide range of psychological and physiological problems. Hypnosis can also be combined with other techniques to promote physical healing. These include visualization, and suggestions directed at body parts or even at cellular tissues (a form of treatment known as cell command therapy). These techniques are still somewhat experimental.

Ericksonian hypnotherapy

One form of hypnotherapy takes its name from Dr. Milton H. Erickson, an American psychiatrist who practiced classic hypnotherapy in the 1950s and 1960s, but also introduced innovative methods for dealing with less straightforward cases. Erickson devised ingenious ways of circumventing reluctance on the part of a client to enter hypnosis and of prompting the acceptance of suggestions. These include the use of metaphor—telling stories with a "hidden message" that the client unconsciously picks up while following the story—and studying individual speech and mannerisms to tailor suggestions to the client's own beliefs and style of expression. Sometimes therapeutic results are achieved through his methods without the client ever feeling that he or she has been formally hypnotized, and this has been called "waking hypnosis."

Attempts have been made by followers of Erickson to draw up systems of indirect suggestion and metaphor based on his practices. Success, however, relies mostly on the individual practitioner's creativity and ingenuity in designing a suitable treatment for a particular client. As with classic hypnotherapy, Ericksonian therapy is often relatively short. The same cautions apply with regard to the advisability of the practitioner being qualified to provide comprehensive psychological support if required.

 Is hypnotherapy compatible with conventional medicine?
Hypnotherapy can be useful in addressing the underlying psychological causes of disorders which are resisting conventional treatment.

 Is a practitioner necessary?
Self-hypnosis is possible, but a practitioner will be required to give guidance on techniques and methods.

EASTERN
THERAPIES

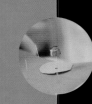

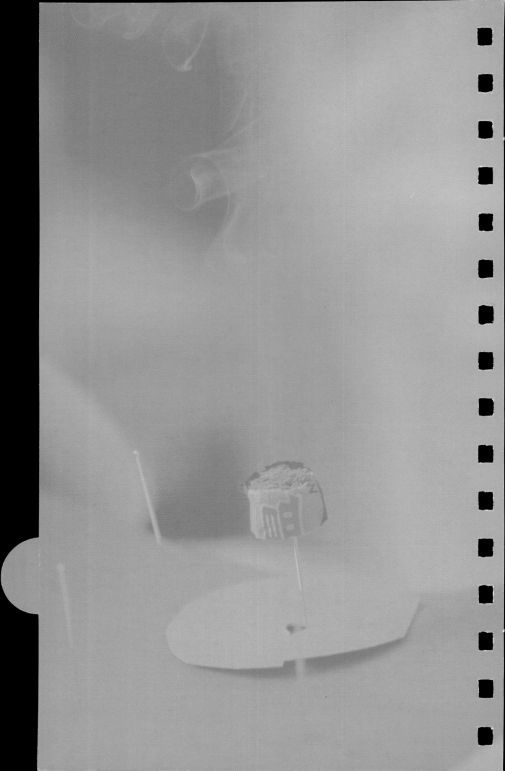

The last decade has seen a huge explosion of interest in therapies from the East, including acupuncture, acupressure, and traditional Chinese medicine, which involves Eastern herbalism and naturopathy, and the Indian system of Ayurveda. These therapies have been in the mainstream of Eastern medicine for centuries. In China, acupuncture, acupressure, and traditional Chinese medicine are considered to be three aspects of one overall healing discipline and are used to treat a person holistically. Ayurveda, based on diet, exercise, and herbalism, is also a holistic therapy. Of all these Eastern therapies, acupuncture is probably the most established in the West, with many qualified practitioners. A reputable, qualified practitioner is essential for all four therapies, although some acupressure can be self-applied.

Ayurveda

Practised in India for more than 3,000 years, Ayurveda (from the Sanskrit "veda," knowledge, and "ayu," life) is the world's most ancient and comprehensive science of natural medicine. Ayurveda provides a wealth of therapies to promote health in both mind and body that have stood the test of time.

In 1980, Maharishi Mahesh Yogi, founder of Transcendental Meditation, gathered the foremost living exponents of Ayurveda to enliven this age-old knowledge in its completeness and original purity. This comprehensively restored system is known as Maharishi Ayurveda.

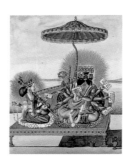

Ayurveda was traditionally believed to have been given by Brahma, the creator, to eliminate human suffering.

Health and the three doshas

Ayurvedic texts describe three aspects to a person: consciousness, mind, and body. For complete health care, you must take care of all three. Maharishi Ayurveda prescribes Transcendental Meditation (TM; see page 30) to enliven awareness of consciousness. This simple mental technique gives direct experience of the silent basis of the three organizing principles, or doshas, that Ayurveda describes as governing mental and physical health, and helps to balance them at their source. Ayurveda also has many different approaches to achieving this balance at the level of mind and body.

The three doshas are called vata, pitta, and kapha. Vata is associated with movement, pitta with metabolism, kapha with solid matter, flesh, and bones. Each dosha has different qualities (see chart on page 150). An imbalance—caused by stress, late nights, wrong food, or other factors—leads to discomfort and even disease. Ayurveda aims to balance the doshas and everyone has a unique proportion of the three that is right for him or her. Knowledge of the doshas can lead to simple remedies. For example, if there is too much pitta dosha, associated with heat, then a cooling activity, food, exercise, or therapy can be prescribed to reduce it.

WILL IT HELP?

• Ayurvedic consultations, educational seminars, and literature help you to monitor your own health, and enable you to recognize and correct the earliest signs of imbalances that can eventually lead to disease.

• Ayurveda recommends natural stress-reduction methods, daily routines, diets, exercises, and other approaches designed to help you gain and maintain ideal health and combat specific ailments. An increasing amount of scientific research is confirming the effectiveness of these traditional approaches.

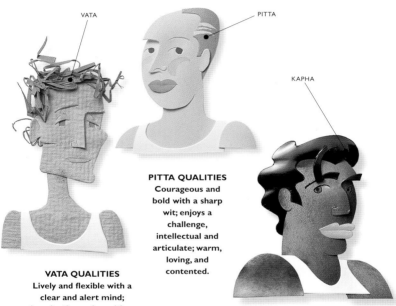

VATA — **PITTA** — **KAPHA**

PITTA QUALITIES
Courageous and bold with a sharp wit; enjoys a challenge, intellectual and articulate; warm, loving, and contented.

VATA QUALITIES
Lively and flexible with a clear and alert mind; imaginative and sensitive; talkative, enthusiastic, and quick to respond.

KAPHA QUALITIES
Compassionate and affectionate with a forgiving nature; emotionally steady and relaxed; methodical with a good memory.

 BENEFITS

• Simple, everyday methods to improve your health problems.
• Reduced stress.
• Prevention of illness through strengthening your healing systems.
• Adds years to life and life to years.

 CAUTION

• Be cautious with your source of Ayurvedic medicines: some imported medicines may contain mercury or other poisonous metals.

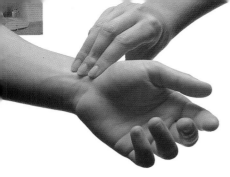

In pulse diagnosis, the three fingers used relate to the three doshas.

Ayurvedic diagnosis

In a consultation, an Ayurvedic doctor will determine the balance of your doshas by taking note of your constitution, pathological state, strength, digestive capacity, age, condition of skin, and other factors. In addition, the doctor will apply nadi vigyan, or pulse diagnosis, which involves feeling your pulse at the wrist, using three fingers. These correspond to the three doshas, and the position, strength, and style of pulse picked up by each finger gives information about the related dosha.

AYURVEDIC RECOMMENDATIONS Based on the diagnosis, an Ayurvedic doctor may make recommendations in the following areas:

• **Behavior** Appropriate advice about daily routines. For example, sleeping late disturbs kapha, while "early to bed" is most important for vata. Different routines may also apply in different seasons. Exercise is important, but should also be according to the balance of the doshas.

• **Food and digestion** Food is medicine in Ayurveda. Inappropriate food, or food of poor quality, can cause disease, while the correct choice of foods can greatly help the healing process. Ayurveda classifies foods as belonging to six taste groups—sweet, sour, salty, pungent, bitter, and astringent. Regularly eating all of the six tastes controls overeating and cravings.

• **Herbal preparations (rasayanas)** While food has a general effect, herbal preparations in Ayurveda are very specific. They act to balance particular functions in the body—such as formation of blood—and to strengthen and rejuvenate. The most gentle, balanced and specific effects are achieved

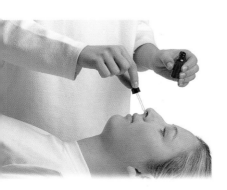

through herbal combinations, and Ayurveda is recognized as having the most complete knowledge of a wide range of herbs. There are no harmful effects from these herbal combinations when prepared in accordance with the ancient texts.

Nasya is a panchakarma treatment that uses oils dropped into the nostrils to treat sinusitis, migraines, facial paralysis, and other head problems.

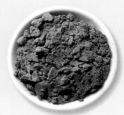

AMRIT KALASH

Maharishi Ayurveda offers two powerful herbal formulas for combating damage introduced in the body by excess free radicals, unstable molecules generated by mental and physical stress, toxic chemicals, and other causes. Maharishi amrit kalash, a traditional combination of 42 Ayurvedic herbs, has been found to be 1,000 times more effective against free radicals than vitamin C and vitamin E, and is the most powerful antioxidant ever discovered. Maharishi amrit kalash, taken as herbal tablets and paste, is designed to work on the most refined level of the body and mind. Regular consumers report reduced stress and fatigue, and increased creativity, energy, and calm.

AMRIT KALASH

• **Purification therapies (panchakarma)**   One of the main purposes of Ayurvedic purification therapy is to cleanse the shrotas (arteries, veins, and lymphatic channels) so that the herbal preparations can have a more powerful effect. Even with Ayurvedic advice, imbalances may still accumulate due to pollution, variations in weather, toxins in food and other factors. Panchakarma is a very sophisticated process of helping the body to remove these imbalances. Panchakarma includes massage treatments with herbalized oils, heat treatments, and various procedures of elimination. Scientific research has found panchakarma to be an effective means of reducing anxiety, depression and fatigue, and increasing energy.

Other Ayurvedic approaches

Ayurveda understands the effects of any experience on our health, and sees that any experience in life can be used to heal. For example, everything picked up by the senses is "ingested," and contributes to balance or imbalance, health or disease. Ayurveda uses sensory approaches to nourish mind and body, including aromatherapy, color therapies, massage, and music therapy, especially through gandharva veda music, which is designed to balance the doshas at different times of day.

Other Vedic sciences that have also been revived in recent decades include how to construct healthy buildings; taking care of wider environmental influences through Vedic astrology; vibration therapy to alleviate chronic disorders using traditional sequences of sound; and strategies to improve the collective health of society.

CHARACTERISTICS OF VATA, PITTA, AND KAPHA		VATA	PITTA ·	KAPHA
	TYPE OF HAIR	DRY	FINE, THINNING, REDDISH, PREMATURELY GRAY	THICK, OILY
	SKIN	DRY, ROUGH	SOFT, RUDDY	OILY, MOIST
	MENTAL ACTIVITY	QUICK MIND, RESTLESS, IMAGINATIVE	SHARP INTELLECT, EFFICIENT, PERFECTIONIST	CALM, STEADY, STABLE
	MEMORY	QUICK TO LEARN, QUICK TO FORGET	GOOD GENERAL MEMORY	GOOD LONG-TERM MEMORY
	WEATHER	AVERSION TO COLD WEATHER	AVERSION TO HOT WEATHER	AVERSION TO DAMP, COOL WEATHER
	SLEEP	INTERRUPTED, LIGHT SLEEP	SOUND, MEDIUM DURATION	SOUND, LONG HEAVY SLEEP
	REACTION TO STRESS	EXCITES EASILY, WORRIED	ANGERS EASILY, IRRITATED, CRITICAL	NOT EASILY RUFFLED, STUBBORN
	BODY SIZE	SMALL FRAME	MEDIUM FRAME	GAIN WEIGHT EASILY
	HUNGER	IRREGULAR	SHARP	CAN EASILY SKIP MEALS
	WALK	QUICK	DETERMINED	SLOW AND STEADY
	MOOD	CHANGE QUICKLY	INTENSE, SLOWLY CHANGING	STEADY, UNCHANGING
	TOTALS			

Identifying your type

You can use the chart above to identify which of the three doshas is most relevant to you. The highest of the three totals indicates the fundamental principle you most need to balance. If two columns have almost the same totals, then you can balance both principles. In the rare case where all three principles are equally present, pay attention to the season: when it's cold and dry, balance vata; when it's hot, balance pitta; when it's cold and damp,

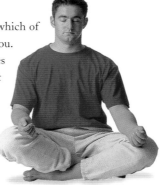

Maintaining a relaxed and positive approach to life assists healing.

balance kapha. When you have identified your type, the vata, pitta, kapha checklist opposite will help you to make simple changes in your diet or daily routine that could help you stay fit and healthy.

	VATA	PITTA	KAPHA
WHEN IN BALANCE	VIBRANT, LIVELY, ENTHUSIASTIC, MIND CLEAR AND ALERT, FLEXIBLE, EXHILARATED, IMAGINATIVE, SENSITIVE, TALKATIVE, QUICK TO RESPOND	WARM, LOVING, CONTENTED, ENJOYS CHALLENGES, STRONG DIGESTION, LUSTROUS COMPLEXION, GOOD CONCENTRATION, ARTICULATE AND PRECISE SPEECH, COURAGEOUS, BOLD, SHARP WIT, INTELLECTUAL	AFFECTIONATE, COMPASSIONATE, FORGIVING, EMOTIONALLY STEADY, RELAXED, SLOW, METHODICAL, GOOD MEMORY, GOOD STAMINA, STABILITY, NATURAL RESISTANCE TO SICKNESS
WHEN OUT OF BALANCE	RESTLESS, UNSETTLED, LIGHT, INTERRUPTED SLEEP, TENDENCY TO OVEREXERT, FATIGUED, CONSTIPATED, ANXIOUS, WORRIED, UNDERWEIGHT	DEMANDING, PERFECTIONIST, TENDENCY TOWARD FRUSTRATION, TENDENCY TOWARD SKIN RASHES, IRRITABLE AND IMPATIENT, PREMATURELY GRAY HAIR, OR EARLY HAIR LOSS	COMPLACENT, DULL OILY SKIN, ALLERGIES, SLOW DIGESTION, LETHARGIC, POSSESSIVE, OVERATTACHED, TENDENCY TO OVERSLEEP, OVERWEIGHT
WHAT AGGRAVATES	IRREGULAR ROUTINE, STAYING UP LATE, IRREGULAR MEALS, COLD DRY WEATHER, EXCESSIVE MENTAL WORK, TOO MUCH BITTER, ASTRINGENT, OR PUNGENT FOOD, TRAVEL, INJURY	EXCESSIVE HEAT OR EXPOSURE TO THE SUN, ALCOHOL, SMOKING, TIME PRESSURE, DEADLINES, EXCESSIVE ACTIVITY, TOO MUCH SPICY, SOUR OR SALTY FOOD, SKIPPING MEALS	EXCESSIVE REST AND OVERSLEEPING, OVER-EATING, INSUFFICIENT EXERCISE, TOO LITTLE VARIETY IN LIFE, HEAVY, UNCTUOUS FOODS, TOO MUCH SWEET, SOUR, OR SALTY FOOD, COLD WET WEATHER.

THE VATA, PITTA, AND KAPHA CHECKLIST

Mind and emotions

Mental states and emotions play an important role in healing. All of the approaches of Maharishi Ayurveda enliven the nourishing qualities of love and respect for our physiology. This in itself is healing, promoting a very positive, healthy attitude rather than the fear of disease, which is detrimental to health. All the strategies of Maharishi Ayurveda help us to recognize what our body is trying to tell us, and to cooperate with our body's natural intelligence to create better health.

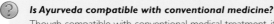

Is Ayurveda compatible with conventional medicine?
Though compatible with conventional medical treatment, it is wise to inform your physician before using any Ayurvedic preparations.

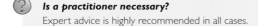

Is a practitioner necessary?
Expert advice is highly recommended in all cases.

Traditional Chinese medicine

Traditional Chinese medicine is holistic on a grand scale. It looks at the mind, the body, and the environment in which an individual lives and works and its underlying rationale is rooted in Chinese views of the creation of the universe and the natural world. It is based on the Daoist (Taoist) philosophy that everything is inter-dependent and mutually interactive, so that body, mind, and spirit are considered not only together but also as part of the same greater life force and cannot be viewed separately.

TCM is both preventive and curative, although the emphasis is on prevention. Its treatments embrace herbal medicine, acupunc-ture, moxibustion, acupressure, diet, meditation, qigong (chi kung) exercises, and feng shui (the art of designing and placing buildings and arranging rooms so that they work in harmony with natural forces). Prevention and cure work together. There is no other way in which TCM could operate.

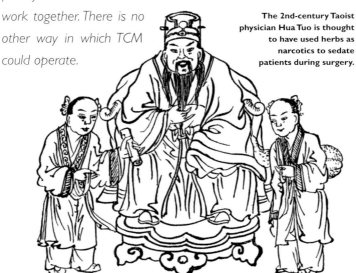

The 2nd-century Taoist physician Hua Tuo is thought to have used herbs as narcotics to sedate patients during surgery.

WILL IT HELP?

• Understanding the principles of TCM and applying them to daily life can help sustain a balanced, healthy body, mind, and spirit. You do not have to wait for the onset of illness to embrace TCM.
• TCM is efficacious in the treatment of many conditions, from stress and psoriasis to duodenal ulcers.
• An increasing number of Western practitioners recognize the effectiveness of acupuncture in the control of pain and other conditions.
• Chinese herbalism can clear conditions, such as acute childhood eczema, with which Western medicine sometimes struggles.

 BENEFITS

• Improved general health in mind, body, and spirit to combat today's stressful and fragmenting pattern of life.
• Broad range of treatments from herbalism to exercise.
• Uses organic instead of drug-based treatments.

 CAUTION

• Certain herbs should not be taken during pregnancy; you should check with your practitioner.
• Some herbs are toxic and should be used with caution under direction.
• Patients with certain liver disorders should not take herbs that are totally contraindicated. Liver function tests are sometimes carried out before herbs are prescribed.
• Patients should not prepare their own remedies except under instruction of a qualified practitioner.
• To be effective, Chinese herbalism needs commitment to the taking of prescribed herbs.

The Chinese approach

Before embarking on traditional Chinese medicine (TCM) it is important to understand that the approach is quite different from that of Western medicine. When the Chinese first encountered Western medicine in the 18th century, a courtier exclaimed that the Western doctors' ideas of illness "were so extraordinary that it appeared as if [they] had come from an inhabitant of another planet." Western practitioners were equally baffled by TCM, and although, today, the two disciplines have drawn closer through mutual learning, they are still very different in approach.

Traditional Chinese practitioners consider disease to be a state of imbalance within the body, caused by imbalances, interactions, or disharmony between individuals and their environment. Consequently the main aim is to preserve or restore a healthy equilibrium: harmonious balance is all. Moreover, from the point of view of TCM changing states of either body or mind can affect the healthy balanced state, and vice versa, so an excessive emotion may cause a bodily illness, or be caused by one.

It is essential that anyone seeking TCM treatment goes to a registered, reputable, qualified practitioner. In the West, there are very few practitioners who offer all the disciplines together and they are usually offered separately. You can find registered practitioners through professional councils or associations. If you find a practitioner through word of mouth, always check their registration. Because treatment is holistic, a qualified practitioner in TCM will not claim to stop you from smoking or guarantee weight loss.

The origins of Chinese medicine can be traced back to the legendary Shen Nong (3494 BCE), discoverer of herbal medicine, and Huangdi (2698–2598 BCE), the Yellow Emperor. The sophisticated practices of TCM were developed and refined from the third century BCE when the *Huangdi Neijing* (*The Yellow Emperor's Classic of Internal Medicine*), one of the seminal texts in the history of Chinese medicine, which contains much earlier material, was written. *Shen Nong Bencaujing* (*Classic of Roots and Herbs of Shen Nong*) was also written down in the third century BCE. By the T'ang dynasty (CE 581–906), physicians knew the cause of goiter and prescribed deer and lamb thyroid as a remedy.

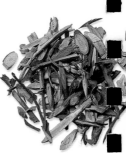

GUI ZHI

CHINESE HERBAL MEDICINE Herbalism, alongside acupuncture, is a fundamental element of TCM. Once a diagnosis is reached the practitioner will prescribe a collection of herbs to restore the body's harmony. The main text on which the written knowledge of Chinese herbalism is based dates from the 16th century when Li Shizhen listed about 2,000 herbs and their uses. It takes great skill to concoct the complex cocktail of functions and qualities in the correct dosage. All parts of plants, from bark to buds, and roots to seeds, are used. The jars of herbs in a TCM dispensary may contain lotus seeds, lily bulb, magnolia buds and bark or watermelon skins.

Each has particular attributes: for example, some herbs have cooling, others warming properties, some are yin and others yang. Not all "herbs" in TCM are plant material either; ground minerals such as kaolin or alum, and parts of animals such as ground shell or bone are used, although alternatives to animal ingredients can often be found. The patient is usually given packages of dry ingredients to take home with instructions on how to boil them with water to make a broth to drink. Pills, powders, and tinctures in alcohol are also prescribed.

Length of treatment varies, but remedies may be taken for several weeks with periodic visits to the practitioner to check progress and adjust dosage as the condition changes. Sometimes, symptoms are exacerbated to begin with, but this is part of the process.

Today, TCM enjoys a growing respect in the West both from patients who have been helped by it, and from the medical profession. There are numerous Western consultants who refer their patients to Chinese herbal practitioners. There are also areas of practice where TCM interconnects with Western medicine. Some Chinese herbs are a source of modern drugs: ephedrine, for example, had its origin in ma huang, a Chinese herb of great antiquity, while licorice, rhubarb, and ginger have all come to be used successfully in Western medicine.

GOU QI ZI

Traditional Chinese medicine sees the human body as part of the natural world. The organs of the body are linked to the five elements of nature, and diagnosis takes account of the characteristics of the relevant element in deciding a treatment.

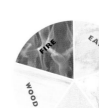
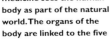

Yin and yang

Yin and yang are the opposing and complementary forces of life, present throughout nature. They are fundamental to TCM, which views the healthy body in terms of a healthy balance between the two. In Chinese thought nothing is purely yin or yang. Each yin object has yang characteristics and vice versa. For example, the liver is a yin organ because it is quite solid, but it has a yang quality in that it influences the flow of qi (chi), or energy, through the body. The stomach is hollow and principally yang, but because it is used for storage it has a yin aspect. The "organs" in Chinese anatomy are groups of closely related physical functions rather than the actual anatomical organs, because Chinese medicine is concerned with function rather than the physical body.

Illness is seen as an excess or deficiency of yin or yang and treatment brings about change that restores balance and harmony. For example, a fever is seen as indicating too much yang, and as the fever breaks and the temperature returns to normal, yang is transformed into yin.

	YIN	YANG
GENERAL	Feminine, earth	Masculine, heavens
QUALITIES	Dark, cold, wet	Light, dry, hot
IN THE BODY	Lower parts, front, inner parts, deeper organs, solid organs	Upper parts, back, outer parts (skin, hair), shallow organs, hollow organs
ORGANS	Yin organs produce and store what are known as the fundamental substances: qi (chi) (life force), blood, jing (energy producing organic development), shen (spirit) fluids (bodily juices).	Yang organs receive, break down, and absorb food that becomes fundamental substances; they also transport and excrete the rest.
CHARACTERISTIC ILLNESS	Dampness invades a body unbalanced by excess yin energy. Symptoms include heavy mucus secretion, discharges. Western diagnosis includes herpes zoster.	Heat invades a body unbalanced by excess yang energy. Symptoms include sudden fevers and hot rashes. Western diagnosis: bacterial infection, such as Streptococcus.

YIN AND YANG IN TRADITIONAL CHINESE MEDICINE

THE FIVE ELEMENTS   Traditional Chinese medicine regards the human body as a microcosm of the universe. It links each of five vital organs—the heart, the liver, the spleen, the lungs, and the kidneys—to one of the five elements: fire, wood, earth, metal, and water. Each of the elements has particular characteristics.
• Fire: dry, hot, ascending, moving
• Wood: growing, flexible, rooted
• Earth: productive, fertile, potential for growth
• Metal: cutting, hard, conducting
• Water: wet, cool, descending, flowing, yielding
The elements all have both yin and yang aspects. They are related to the body/emotions and the natural world in a complex way. The organs are associated with the attributes of the five elements (see table below): this is significant for diagnosis and treatment. For example, wood symbolizes the active process of growth. It is associated with Spring, and with the liver and the gallbladder, the active regulators of the rest of the body.

ELEMENT	WOOD	FIRE	EARTH	METAL	WATER
SEASON	Spring	Summer	late Summer	Autumn	Winter
DIRECTION	East	South	Center	West	North
CLIMATE	Wind	Heat	Damp	Dry	Cold
COLOR	Blue/green	Red	Yellow	White	Black
TASTE	Sour	Bitter	Sweet	Pungent	Salty
SMELL	Rancid	Burnt	Fragrant	Rotting	Putrid
YIN ORGAN	Liver	Heart	Spleen	Lungs	Kidney
YANG ORGAN	Gall-bladder	Small intestine	Stomach	Large intestine	Bladder
ORIFICE	Eyes	Tongue	Mouth	Nose	Ears
TISSUE	Tendons	Blood vessels	Flesh/muscles	Skin	Bones
EMOTION	Anger	Joy	Pensiveness	Grief	Fear
VOICE	Shout	Laugh	Sing	Weep	Groan

THE FIVE ELEMENTS AND THEIR ATTRIBUTES

CHI (QI)

The notion of chi (qi) (pronounced "chee") is at the root of traditional Chinese medicine. Everything in the universe is composed of chi, which is translated as "energy" or "life force." Chi flows through the universe, and through its microcosm, the human body. The flow of chi through the energy meridians in the body is fundamental to good health. TCM practitioners monitor the levels and flow of chi, and often use acupuncture to remove obstructions and regulate its flow.

Diagnosis

Western patients new to traditional Chinese medicine are often surprised by the length of time given to diagnosis. An initial consultation can take more than an hour and many questions can seem irrelevant. It seems odd to be asked about colors and seasons when you have a stomach ache. But TCM diagnosis is a complex examination of the whole individual and will lead to a holistic remedy.

Energy flows through a network of meridians or channels. These channels connect the organs to each other in various ways, and also allow each internal organ to communicate with a surface organ on the body: heart to tongue, liver to eyes, spleen to mouth, lungs to nose, kidney to ear. This idea is essential to diagnosis in TCM. Along the body's meridian network, there are points where the flow of chi is accessible to outside (medical) intervention. (These are the acupuncture points.)

Practitioners use four methods—looking, hearing and smelling, questioning, and touching—to reach a diagnosis. Looking involves observing weight, body language, color and general appearance of hair, face and skin, so it's best not to wear makeup to a TCM session. The state of the tongue is crucial in the looking part of diagnosis. In hearing and smelling a practitioner can tell much from the quality of the voice, the amount a patient talks, and the way in which an individual breathes. Bodily odors can also give clues to illness, so it's important not to use perfumed soaps and sprays before a consultation. Answers to questions give insight

The initial TCM consultation can take a long time, but it gives the practitioner a complete picture on which to base a diagnosis and suggest treatment.

into all aspects of the patient's spiritual, mental, and physical life, as well as specific symptoms. Body temperature, moisture, and pain are important in diagnostic touching. However, the most important aspect is pulse-taking. Examination of the pulse is complex. The Chinese have identified about 200 pulses to be checked in diagnosis, and three different pressures to be used—light, medium and heavy—in determining the character of the pulse. Pulse descriptions can be poetic: "sharp as a hook," "fine as a hair." "dead as a rock," "smooth as a flowing stream," "sharp as a bird's beak," and "the front crooked and the back delayed."

Is TCM compatible with conventional medicine?
TCM can complement conventional medicine, and some Western practitioners refer patients to Chinese herbalists.

Is a practitioner necessary?
The complexity of TCM and the importance of diagnosis makes a practitioner essential.

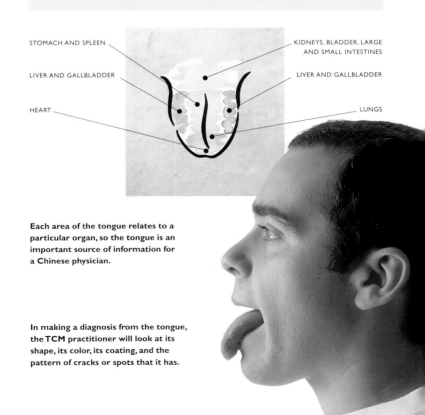

STOMACH AND SPLEEN

KIDNEYS, BLADDER, LARGE AND SMALL INTESTINES

LIVER AND GALLBLADDER

LIVER AND GALLBLADDER

HEART

LUNGS

Each area of the tongue relates to a particular organ, so the tongue is an important source of information for a Chinese physician.

In making a diagnosis from the tongue, the TCM practitioner will look at its shape, its color, its coating, and the pattern of cracks or spots that it has.

Acupuncture

Acupuncture is a form of therapy that involves the insertion of fine needles into selected points in the body. It is generally regarded as having originated in China some 3,000 years ago, although acupuncture-like techniques have developed independently in several other communities around the world. Indeed, the earliest indication of the use of such techniques comes from Europe and is revealed by the study of the Tyrolean Ice Man, whose recently discovered remains date back over 5,000 years.

In the East acupuncture grew up as an integral part of Chinese medicine within its framework of Chinese philosophy, and it is still practiced within this traditional framework today. However, there are increasing numbers of healthcare workers throughout the world training in what has become known as Western medical acupuncture. This combines the practice of acupuncture with Western medical theory, techniques, and treatment, and this is a good example of the way that traditional therapies are being adopted in the West.

The theories of yin and yang lie at the root of Chinese medicine. These opposing, yet interdependent forces must be in balance for good health.

WILL IT HELP?

• Acupuncture is particularly useful in treating muscular aches and pains anywhere in the body.
• Other painful conditions, such as headaches, migraines, sinusitis, irritable bowel syndrome, and menstrual problems, can respond very well.
• Acupuncture treatment is worth trying for any painful condition.
• Selected nonpainful complaints, such as hay fever, digestive problems, gynecological problems, and bladder irritation, can be managed effectively in some cases.
• In general some 70 percent of patients seem to benefit from the use of acupuncture.

 BENEFITS

• Reduces the need for painkillers and other drugs.
• Helps to relax tense muscles and promotes stress relief.
• Improves sleep pattern.

 CAUTION

• Always seek a suitably trained registered practitioner.
• Always get a doctor's opinion before seeking treatment for unexplained symptoms or problems.
• Always tell the practitioner, before treatment, about any heart valve problem, bleeding tendency (including use of anticoagulants), or suspected pregnancy.

Prehistoric acupuncture needles were made of stone. Today's needles are much finer than hypodermic needles and if inserted correctly are barely felt.

How acupuncture works

Over the last 25 years, scientists in both the East and the West have been investigating how acupuncture works. There now seems no doubt that its beneficial effects are produced through stimulation of nerves at the site of needle insertion. This results in the release of endorphins within the nervous system. Endorphins are one group of the body's naturally occurring chemical messengers, and are best known for their powerful painkilling effects, but they have other less recognized functions, such as boosting the immune system.

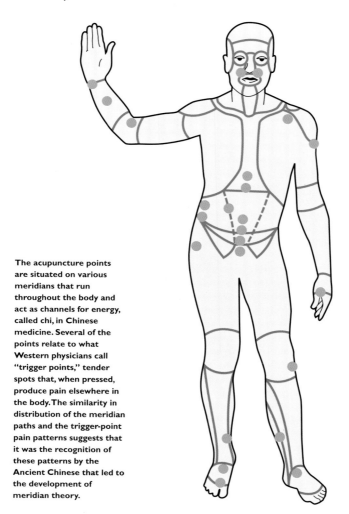

The acupuncture points are situated on various meridians that run throughout the body and act as channels for energy, called chi, in Chinese medicine. Several of the points relate to what Western physicians call "trigger points," tender spots that, when pressed, produce pain elsewhere in the body. The similarity in distribution of the meridian paths and the trigger-point pain patterns suggests that it was the recognition of these patterns by the Ancient Chinese that led to the development of meridian theory.

Acupuncture is particularly useful for treating muscular aches and pains. If you can find a tender point which, when pressed on, reproduces your pain or other symptoms, it is very likely that acupuncture will effect a cure or substantial benefit. If you suffer with headaches, related tender points may be found in the muscles of the neck and shoulders. If you have pain running down the arm, related tender points may be found in the muscles of the shoulder girdle; and if you have pain running down the leg, related tender points may be found in the muscles of the hip girdle. Pain and "pins and needles" in the arm or leg are often misdiagnosed as a "trapped nerve."

An experienced acupuncturist will often be able to trace such a problem to a "trigger point" source that may be located some distance away. Such trigger points can be treated quickly and easily with an acupuncture needle.

Modern approaches

Broadly speaking, practitioners take either a Western medical approach or an Eastern traditional approach to the use of acupuncture. Doctors and other healthcare workers who are trained in orthodox medicine use acupuncture as one of a number of therapies available to them, and will make an orthodox diagnosis before deciding on which therapy to use.

Practitioners who use the Eastern approach make an assessment based on the theoretical movement of energy around the body. This energy is said to travel around the body in specific nonphysical channels known as meridians. The assessment is made by taking a history, and examining the tongue and taking the pulse in several ways at both wrists. There is clearly an advantage in having an orthodox diagnosis before embarking on treatment, as the effective benefits of acupuncture in treating pain can mask the symptoms of serious disease. However, the Eastern approach has the benefit of allowing several apparently unconnected symptoms to be viewed as part of the same "disharmony" of energy flow, and the thought that all of their problems can be brought together in this way is comforting to some individuals.

THE COLOR OF THE TONGUE CAN BE REVEALING

Tongue diagnosis is an important part of the Eastern approach.

Acupuncture points

No matter which approach is used, the needles will still affect the body in similar ways, and there is often considerable overlap in the points used. This is particularly the case when considering muscular and soft tissue pain. The Western practitioner will examine the subject carefully for "trigger points" at the source of the pain and treat these. The Eastern approach may involve feeling along the course of a meridian, along which acupuncture points are located, until a tender point is found. Trigger points and acupuncture points often correspond, and the pain pattern produced by trigger points frequently appears to match the path of the corresponding meridian. It is perhaps no surprise to find that acupuncture is most effective in circumstances where the two approaches overlap, such as in the treatment of simple muscular aches and pains.

Some people are put off by the thought of having needles inserted through their skin, perhaps because of past experience of injections. Acupuncture needles are much finer than those used for injections, and the ends have a different shape; consequently, if acupuncture needles are inserted quickly through the skin, the sensation is barely perceptible. Having passed through the skin, the needle may be advanced into deeper tissue, where the most frequent sensation is one of dullness or numbness. This is traditionally thought to represent "energy" accumulating around the needle, and indicates that it is probably correctly sited for optimal effect.

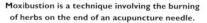
Moxibustion is a technique involving the burning of herbs on the end of an acupuncture needle.

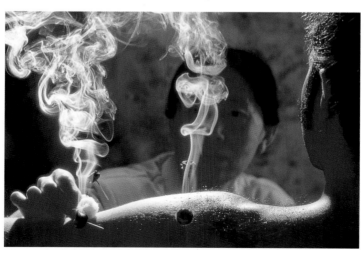

OTHER FORMS OF ACUPUNCTURE

• Moxibustion involves burning moxa, the pith of the herb *Artemisia vulgaris* (mugwort), at or near acupuncture points in order to regulate the flow of chi. Pieces of moxa can be placed on needles inserted into the skin, or alternatively a moxa stick is held close to the skin. Moxibustion to the acupuncture point BL67 on the small toe has been shown to turn babies in the womb from the breech position to the normal head-down position, allowing a safer natural delivery.

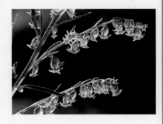

***Artemisia vulgaris* (mugwort)**

• Ear acupuncture, or auriculotherapy, can be useful for painful and non-painful conditions, as an alternative or in addition to body acupuncture, and it may be useful in the treatment of drug and nicotine dependence.

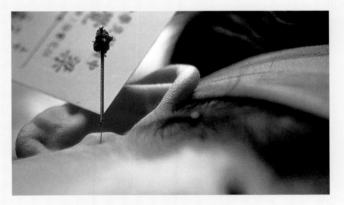

Auriculotherapy helps control pain.

• Laser therapy—laser treatment to acupuncture points—is used by some practitioners as an alternative to needling.

• Electroacupuncture is a powerful and effective form of therapy that was first developed for pain relief during surgery. It is particularly useful in the treatment of chronic pain, but has many further applications, and has been used successfully to enhance wound healing. Electroacupuncture should be avoided by patients who have a pacemaker.

• There is increasing interest in acupuncture in the veterinary profession, whose clientele are thought less likely to respond to a placebo.

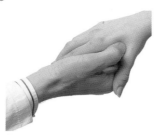

You can relieve pain from headaches or toothaches by pressing on LI4 in the web between thumb and forefinger

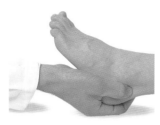

Pressure on the bladder meridian in the heel can alleviate bedwetting.

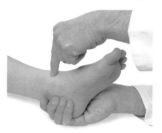

Points on the spleen meridian may also help with this problem.

Acupressure

Acupressure is a weaker form of stimulation than acupuncture, although acupressure actually developed first, and it is still widely practiced in China. It also forms part of the Japanese pressure therapy, Shiatsu. There are some acupuncture therapists who use the technique alongside acupuncture, but most practitioners take the view that, although it may offer some short-term relief of symptoms, its benefits are not as long-lasting in treating disorders as those of acupuncture proper.

Acupressure uses manual pressure on the acupuncture points instead of inserting needles into them. Pressure can be applied with the fingers or thumbs, or with a blunt instrument. Acupressure is a good self-help technique, since it requires little specialist training, and it is also useful for treating children who may be alarmed at the idea of needles. Charts showing the location of useful acupoints are available. You should not use self-treatment if you are pregnant since some acupoints should not be stimulated during pregnancy

Is acupuncture compatible with conventional medicine?

Both Eastern and Western approaches can be used in conjunction with conventional medical treatment.

Is a practitioner necessary?

Yes. Acupuncture should only be carried out by properly trained and qualified practitioners, although acupressure can be self-administered without any danger.

MANIPULATIVE THERAPIES

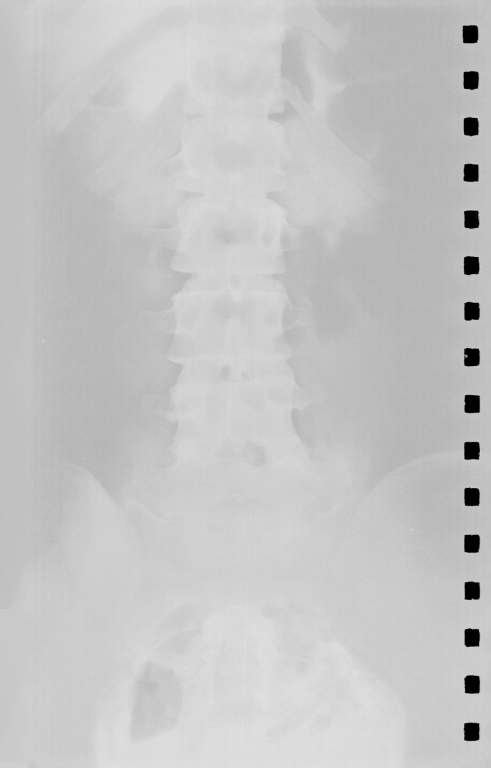

Concentration on the mechanics of the human body has led to the development of two manipulative therapies which are enjoying increasing success and popularity, and gradual acceptance by the medical establishment. Osteopathy and chiropractic are now used by many people, especially to deal with back pain. The therapies are related: osteopathy was devised by American doctor Andrew Taylor Still and chiropractic by his pupil, Daniel Palmer. Osteopathy identifies and deals with the structural malfunctions and misalignments that prevent the body from getting on with the job of healing itself. Chiropractic pays more attention to manipulation of the spine. Various offshoots have developed from both disciplines: cranial osteopathy and McTimoney chiropractic are probably the best known. Both therapies are very much a hands-on experience, and a qualified practitioner is essential.

Chiropractic

The first chiropractic treatment (known as adjustment) was given by the Canadian Daniel David Palmer in 1895. Palmer, a student of anatomy and physiology, theorized that if the spine is the path through which the central nervous system sends the brain's messages, then any restriction of the spine owing to injury or poor posture could interfere with those messages, causing pain or disease. He tested his theory on janitor Harvey Lillard who, while working in cramped conditions 17 years before, had felt something "give" in his spine, after which he went deaf. Palmer found that one of Lillard's vertebrae was misaligned. He adjusted the vertebra whereupon Lillard's hearing was discovered to have improved dramatically.

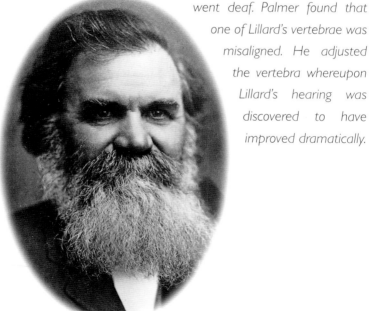

After successfully treating his janitor's spine, **Canadian Daniel David Palmer** moved to Davenport in Iowa. There he continued to develop the principles of chiropractic, establishing the first chiropractic school.

Chiropractors manipulate joints and muscles to stimulate the body into healing itself.

WILL IT HELP?

- A Medical Research Council trial found chiropractic to be more effective than hospital out-patient treatment for low back pain.
- Chiropractic can keep arthritic joints mobile, reducing pain and helping to slow further degeneration.
- The therapy can be used on joints affected by repetitive strain injury (RSI) to minimize stress on muscles, nerves, and tendons.
- It can relieve neck pain, whiplash injuries, and many types of headache.
- As well as treating sports injuries, chiropractors can carry out preseason checks to help athletes maintain optimum performance.
- Treatment is individually tailored to each patient, and is therefore safe and suitable for pregnant women, babies, and children.
- Successful treatment of period pain, infantile colic, "glue ear," digestive problems, chronic fatigue syndrome, and other disorders is frequently reported.

 BENEFITS

- Relieves pain and improves general mobility.
- Reduces spinal nerve stress, allowing the body's own healing processes to improve and maintain health.
- Suitable for everyone.

 CAUTION

- Before undergoing treatment, check that your practitioner is fully qualified and insured.

What is chiropractic?

Chiropractic specializes in the diagnosis, treatment, and overall management of conditions that are a result of mechanical dysfunction of the joints and muscles and their effects on the nervous system. We all know that the body is capable of healing itself and we take the rapid healing of cuts, bruises, and broken bones for granted. If, however, whether through accident or lifestyle, a joint or vertebra loses its normal mobility, this can affect the nervous system, and interfere with the natural healing process. This in turn can lead to pain, discomfort, or even disease. Chiropractors restore full function to the affected joint, allowing the body to return more rapidly to its normal level of health.

Consultation and diagnosis

A chiropractor begins a first consultation by asking questions about your symptoms, medical history, lifestyle, and posture. You will then be fully examined with the use of standard neurological and orthopedic tests. The chiropractor may, if necessary to aid the diagnosis, also take or order xrays. Some practitioners are also qualified in applied kinesiology, which is a method of muscle testing that can pinpoint imbalances and weaknesses throughout the body.

A full training in differential diagnosis and radiology ensures that if a chiropractor's examination identifies underlying disease, or a condition for which chiropractic is inappropriate, he or she will immediately refer you to a medical physician or consultant. Chiropractors do not prescribe drugs or use surgical procedures.

Once the chiropractor has identified the cause of your symptoms, and explained it fully to you, treatment begins. It involves the use of gentle hand movements known as adjustments directed at the joints that are under stress, and the muscles surrounding them. Exact treatment techniques, and the number and frequency of visits, vary according to the needs of the individual, making chiropractic appropriate for everyone, from the newborn to the athlete, and from pregnant women to the elderly.

Often, an adjustment will involve a very rapid "thrusting" action that moves the two surfaces of a joint apart. This causes a change of pressure within the joint space, and the noise that sometimes results is the characteristic sound of a bubble of gas popping. This sound has no other signif-

icance and the experience is not painful. Following treatment, the chiropractor may recommend the use of ice or heat, give lifestyle and dietary
advice, and prescribe appropriate rehabilitation exercises.

Although you do not need a physician's referral to visit a chiropractor,
some physicians do purchase chiropractic treatment for their patients on
national health schemes. Many health insurance companies now include
chiropractic among their benefits.

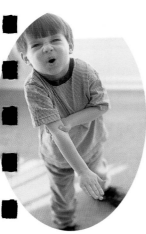
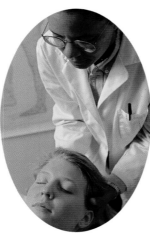

**Xrays are often used
to help the chiropractor
make a diagnosis.**

**Even babies and young
children respond
to chiropractic. Injury
to a joint may affect
the nervous system,
slowing the healing
process. Chiropractic
reverses this.**

**Manipulating the cervical
vertebrae of the spine
can ease a whiplash injury
caused by a car crash.**

RESEARCH

• In 1989 a study in Denmark revealed that when spinal adjustments were
given to 316 infants suffering from colic, 94 percent were relieved of
symptoms within two weeks.

• In 1994 the Agency for Health Care Policy and Research recommended
manipulation as the preferred form of treatment for low back pain.

• In 1995 the follow-up of a Medical Research Council trial concluded that
patients with low back pain treated with chiropractic derive more benefit
and long-term satisfaction than those treated by hospitals.

• In 1996 and 1999 the Royal College of General Practitioners issued
guidelines for GPs recommending manipulative treatment for low back
pain and stating that the risks of manipulation are very low in skilled hands.

• In 1997 a trial at the University of Odense in Denmark showed
chiropractic as an effective treatment for neck-related headaches.

Preventive treatment and self-help

It is not possible to adjust your own joints; you are more likely to "pop" the wrong joint since movement in the affected one will be restricted. However, while it is essential to see a qualified practitioner for treatment, you can help yourself by paying attention to your posture, adhering to the exercise program your chiropractor gives you, and following a healthy lifestyle.

Just as regular visits to the dentist can identify and treat signs of decay before you experience any pain, regular checkups with a chiropractor can highlight restrictions in joint movement before any symptoms appear. This is especially important in babies and children, whose still-growing bones can be affected by the rough and tumble of their lives, while symptoms may not appear until their teens or even later. If the symptoms that brought you to a chiropractor have been caused by your lifestyle—perhaps a sports activity, or a working environment that cannot be changed or avoided—he or she may recommend regular checkups or treatment to prevent any future recurrence of the problem.

During pregnancy it's wise to attend regular checkups to monitor the condition of the joints and muscles.

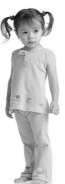

Young children also benefit from regular checks. Childhood damage to joints or muscles may not appear until later in life.

Training and qualifications

Common international standards of education have been achieved through a network of accrediting agencies that began with the U.S. Council on Chiropractic Education (CCE), recognized by the U.S. Office of Education since 1974. There are 16 chiropractic colleges in the U.S. accredited by the CCE.

Entrance requirements vary according to country, but are a minimum of two years university credits in qualifying subjects in North America. The chiropractic college undergraduate program has a minimum of four fulltime academic years, followed by postgraduate clinical training. Postgraduate specialties include chiropractic sciences, orthopedics, radiology, rehabilitation, and sports chiropractic. There are approximately 50,000 chiropractors in the United States.

• Pain is a warning sign: do not ignore it.

• Make frequent, small changes in your sitting or standing position whenever you are sitting or standing still.

• Sit on firm but cushioned chairs with a comfortable backrest.

• Adjust the driving seat of your car properly.

• Climb up rather than reach up.

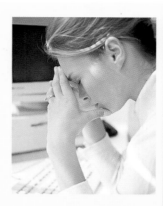

GOLDEN RULES FOR HEALTHY JOINTS

• Don't work too long in one position—take a short break regularly.

• Never bend when you can kneel or squat.

• Do not cough or sneeze in a bent position.

• When lifting a heavy weight prepare yourself properly, remembering to bend your knees, and do not twist.

• Distribute heavy weights equally when carrying.

• Never sit, stoop, or bend for prolonged periods.

• For sleeping use one pillow and a good supportive mattress.

• Never exercise without a warm-up and cool-down.

• If you have back pain, do not stay in bed for prolonged periods: bed-rest can slow your recovery.

• If you can, avoid doing your heaviest or most prolonged work during the first two hours of your day.

 Is chiropractic compatible with conventional medicine?
Yes. Many general practitioners (physicians) and consultants refer their patients for chiropractic treatment, and indeed, many are chiropractic patients themselves.

 Is a practitioner necessary?
It is essential to see a qualified practitioner for treatment, but you can help to take care of your joints with good posture and exercise.

Osteopathy

Osteopathy is a system of healing related to manipulation and bonesetting, which have their roots in the earliest medical history. It was founded in the US at the end of the 19th century by the physician Andrew Taylor Still and is based on the philosophy that physiological structure and function are intimately interrelated. Still developed osteopathy after tragically losing two of his children to spinal meningitis. He came to believe that the system of an individual with the correct body alignment and posture would function optimally, so they would not be affected by disease. The practice of osteopathy has since been developed by such practitioners as Fryette, who advanced the concept of the "total lesion" to include nutrition, lifestyle, and psychosomatic factors, and Sutherland, who started the practice of cranial osteopathy.

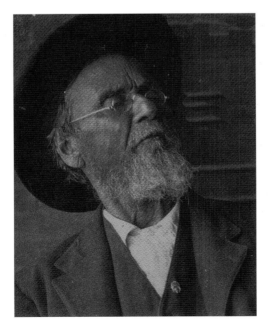

Andrew Taylor Still trained as an engineer before turning to medicine and becoming an army surgeon. He came to believe that by adjusting the body's framework, it could be stimulated to heal itself.

WILL IT HELP?

• Osteopathy is not a quick fix, nor a cure for a list of specific ailments. It is, however, an extremely effective form of treatment which can benefit a wide range of conditions and which involves the patient in the healing process.

• Treatment can help to reduce the effects of stress-related conditions.

• A practitioner is needed to apply the treatment, but without the support of the patient, and the patient's willingness to follow advice, progress will be difficult.

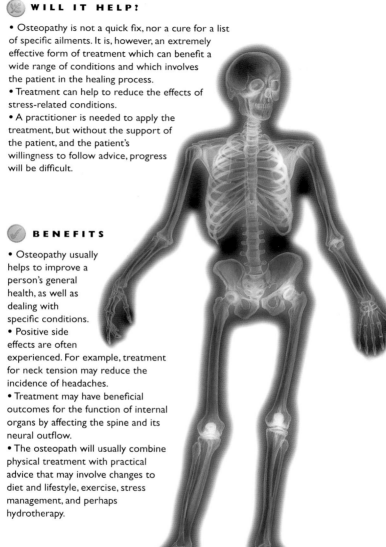

 BENEFITS

• Osteopathy usually helps to improve a person's general health, as well as dealing with specific conditions.

• Positive side effects are often experienced. For example, treatment for neck tension may reduce the incidence of headaches.

• Treatment may have beneficial outcomes for the function of internal organs by affecting the spine and its neural outflow.

• The osteopath will usually combine physical treatment with practical advice that may involve changes to diet and lifestyle, exercise, stress management, and perhaps hydrotherapy.

 CAUTION

• Osteopathy is not a self-help therapy and treatment should be received only from a qualified and registered practitioner.

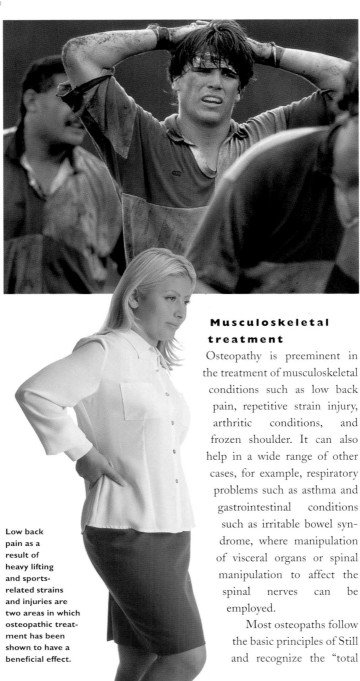

Musculoskeletal treatment

Osteopathy is preeminent in the treatment of musculoskeletal conditions such as low back pain, repetitive strain injury, arthritic conditions, and frozen shoulder. It can also help in a wide range of other cases, for example, respiratory problems such as asthma and gastrointestinal conditions such as irritable bowel syndrome, where manipulation of visceral organs or spinal manipulation to affect the spinal nerves can be employed.

Most osteopaths follow the basic principles of Still and recognize the "total

Low back pain as a result of heavy lifting and sports-related strains and injuries are two areas in which osteopathic treatment has been shown to have a beneficial effect.

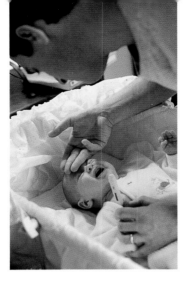

Cranial osteopathy is based on the idea that the cerebrospinal fluid that supports the brain flows with a certain rhythm. Osteopaths believe that disruptions to this rhythm might be connected to infant colic and other childhood disorders, and gentle manipulation of the skull can help restore a balanced rhythm.

lesion" concept of Fryette, which is based on the finding that any disease is likely to be a composite of many factors, which may include a postural anomaly, a dietetic influence, a stress factor, and an infective agent. Osteopathy also views the human system as a totally integrated and interdependent whole, so that if one physiological system is compromised all systems will be correspondingly compromised to a greater or lesser extent. A patient with a respiratory problem, for example, will also suffer changes in the circulatory, excretory, and digestive systems, all of which may show signs or symptoms of distress. If, in this case, a symptom of distress in the excretory system is treated on its own, then the real cause of the problem is not being addressed. This simple example illustrates the need to find the cause of the disease and focus on this while treating the whole person.

Osteopathy is based on the principle of structure governing function, whether it be at the gross anatomical level or at the cellular, biochemical level. The principal aim of the osteopath is to help to restore the body's structural balance in order to obtain functional integrity. Treatment must be practitioner-led and it is not feasible to treat oneself by osteopathy. However, the patient will be given advice by the practitioner on ways to aid and support recovery.

Traditionally osteopaths treat the musculoskeletal and visceral systems. More recently the use of cranial osteopathy has blossomed and many practitioners also use this technique, which involves subtle pressure applied to the skull and suboccipital structures at the base of the skull to influence the body as a whole. This technique is especially useful for children and the frail and elderly. Osteopaths employ soft tissue and joint manipulation and some also use equipment such as electrotherapy, ultrasound, and therapeutic light.

Treatment by an osteopath

When a patient visits an osteopathic practice for the first time a complete case history is normally taken, followed by a physical examination and clinical screen, including a structural/postural examination, appropriate orthopedic (spine and joints) tests, tendon reflexes, and functional tests, taking blood pressure, and heart, lung and retinal examination. The patient has to undress to underwear so that the osteopath can also observe anatomical alignment and skin color and texture.

Treatment may involve soft-tissue manipulation and joint manipulation and advice on therapeutic exercises, together possibly with dietary and lifestyle advice and stress management guidelines. The first consultation is likely to be an hour in length, with treatment. Follow-up treatment is likely to be at weekly intervals—sometimes more frequently at first—and these visits are likely to be 30 minutes. The patient may feel tired after treatment, but some benefit is usually felt immediately.

Osteopaths may work with other healthcare practitioners, such as naturopaths, acupuncturists, homeopaths, herbalists, and chiropractors. All these distinct therapies are compatible and all have the overriding objective of helping the patient both by treatment and by educating him or her to understand how best to reestablish and maintain health. Many osteopaths are also naturopaths and some are acupuncturists or herbalists.

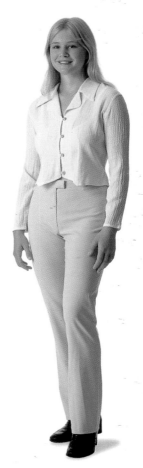

Osteopathy seeks to restore the body's structural integrity

Is osteopathy compatible with conventional medicine?
Osteopathy is compatible with conventional treatments, and some GPs are also trained osteopaths.

Is a practitioner necessary?
Yes. It is not possible to practice osteopathy as a self-help technique, and so a qualified osteopath is essential.

YOU AND

YOUR NEEDS

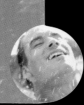

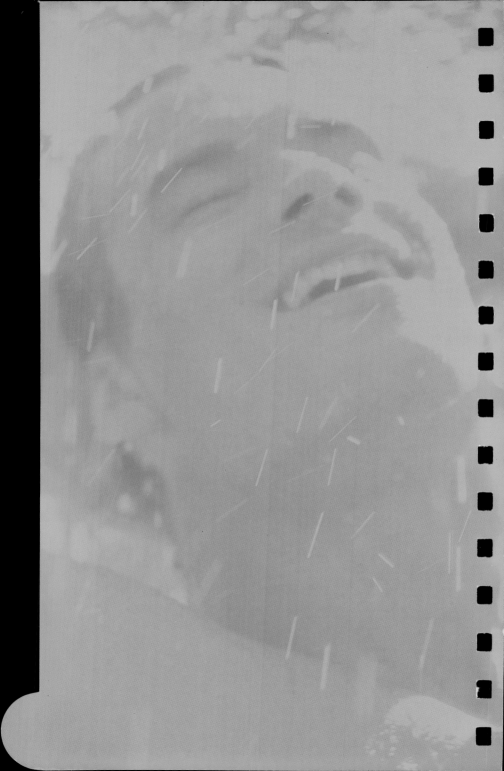

This section brings it all together. A checklist of ailments shows which will respond best to which therapy and a first-aid chart shows you how the therapies can be useful in domestic emergencies. The glossary introduces and defines the more unusual terms that complementary therapists might use. A comprehensive list of addresses directs you to organizations and institutes where you can find out more, and there is also a listing of all the contributors to this book.

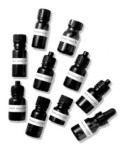

Treating common ailments

Many of the therapies featured in this directory are holistic, meaning that they treat the whole person rather than addressing specific ailments, symptoms, or conditions. However, there are some conditions that benefit very directly from particular types of complementary therapy, and this table lists some common ailments and the therapies that are appropriate.

Some therapies have been listed beside every ailment, for example, healing and color therapy. These are types of energy medicine, and address imbalances of mind, body, and spirit that can arise from, or be the cause of, specific symptoms. Hence, any kind of physical or mental disorder could benefit from treatment. Ayurveda, osteopathy, and naturopathy have been omitted from the table because these therapies are person-centered and treatment depends on the complete picture of symptoms that a patient presents to the practitioner.

IMMUNE SYSTEM
INFECTION
ALLERGIES
FEVER
INFLUENZA
SORE THROAT
SHINGLES
HERPES SIMPLEX
HEAD AND THROAT
RESPIRATORY SYSTEM
PHLEGM
COMMON COLD
COUGHS AND BRONCHITIS
HAY FEVER
SINUSITIS
ASTHMA
HICCUPS
HEART AND CIRCULATORY SYSTEM
ANEMIA
CHILBLAINS
VARICOSE VEINS
RESTLESS LEGS
MUSCLES, BONES, AND JOINTS
BACK PAIN
ARTHRITIS
OSTEOARTHRITIS
OSTEOPOROSIS
RHEUMATISM
CRAMPS
RSI
NERVOUS SYSTEM
NEURALGIA
HEADACHES
MIGRAINES
FATIGUE
CHRONIC FATIGUE SYNDROME
STRESS
INSOMNIA
SEASONAL AFFECTIVE DISORDER (SAD)

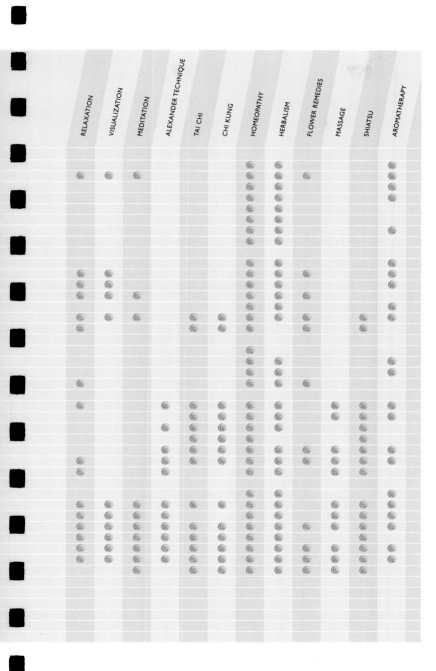

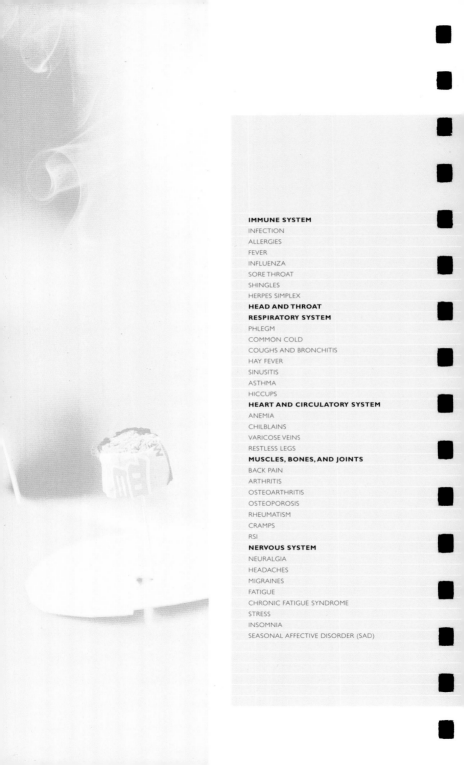

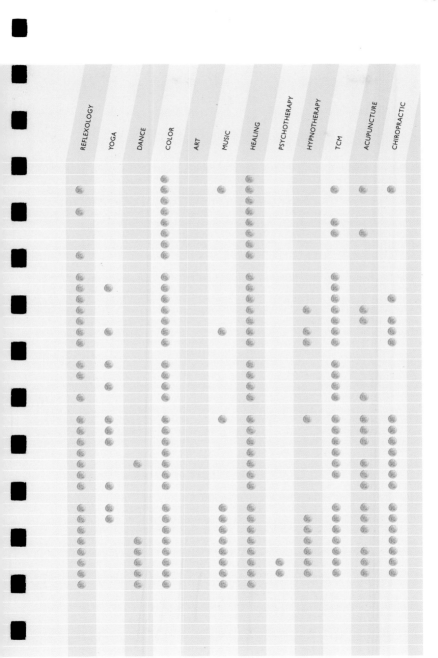

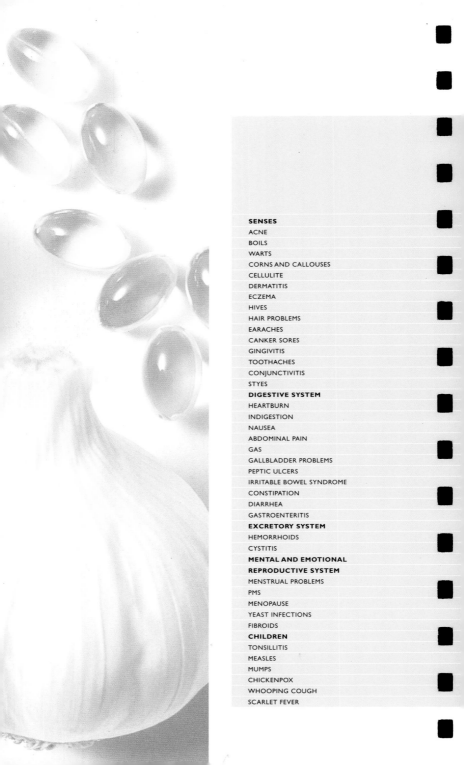

	RELAXATION	VISUALIZATION	MEDITATION	ALEXANDER TECHNIQUE	TAI CHI	CHI KUNG	HOMEOPATHY	HERBALISM	FLOWER REMEDIES	MASSAGE	SHIATSU	AROMATHERAPY

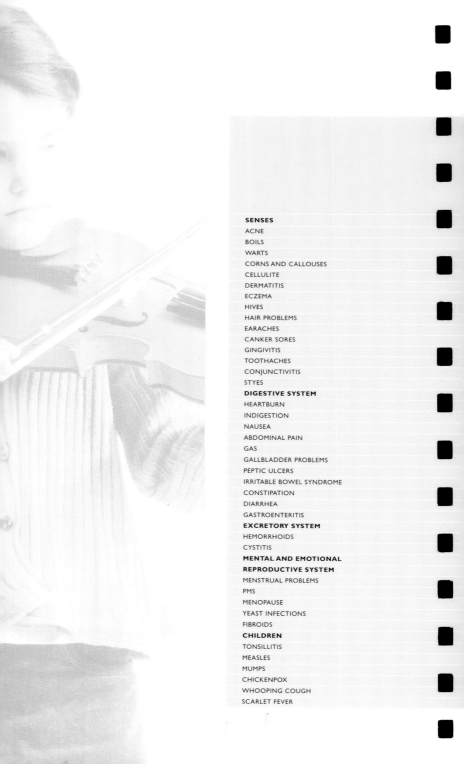

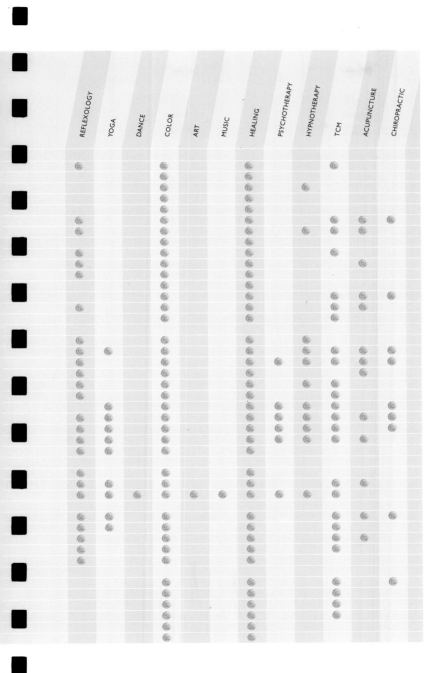

First aid

Some of the therapies in this book are appropriate for treating minor injuries and accidents. There are numerous herbal, homeopathic, and aromatherapeutic remedies available to relieve minor aches and pains, while flower remedies will help to calm someone after an accident. Detailed here are a few common first-aid treatments. Serious emergencies should always be dealt with by qualified medical professionals.

Cuts

Cuts should be cleaned and covered with an adhesive dressing when the bleeding has stopped.

AROMATHERAPY Clean the cut using a bowl of warm water to which you have added 5 drops of lavender or tea tree oil.

HOMEOPATHY Hypericum 30c can be used to relieve the pain of a cut finger.

HERBAL REMEDIES Creams containing calendula, St. John's wort, or chamomile can be used to soothe cuts.

Sunburn

Susceptibility to sunburn varies from person to person, and there is the obvious danger of skin cancer resulting from excessive exposure to the sun. Severe sunburn with blisters should be referred to a physician.

AROMATHERAPY A cool bath with peppermint or lavender essential oil will ease a mild sunburn.

HOMEOPATHY Belladonna 6c or Glonoine 6c will relieve headaches caused by sun exposure.

HERBAL REMEDIES An infusion of St. John's wort oil can be applied to ease a sunburn.

Burns

Burns are often accompanied by shock. For small burns hold the affected area under cold running water until the pain diminishes. Never use butter or oil on burns. Severe burns need urgent hospital treatment.

AROMATHERAPY Neat lavender oil relieves pain, after holding the burn under running water.

HOMEOPATHY Arnica 30c is a good remedy to use after any trauma.

HERBAL REMEDIES Minor burns can be soothed with a compress soaked in a cool infusion of chickweed, St. John's wort, calendula or plantain.

FLOWER REMEDIES Four drops of Rescue Remedy on the tongue will help to relieve shock.

Bruises

Bruises result from bleeding below the skin after a blow.

AROMATHERAPY Put two drops of lavender and two drops of chamomile into a bowl of hot water, and two drops of each into a bowl of cold water. Soak a facecloth in each bowl, and apply the hot and cold cloths alternately to the bruise.

HOMEOPATHY Arnica 30c is a good remedy for bruises and aches. Bellis perennis 30c is effective for more severe bruising.

HERBAL REMEDIES A cold compress soaked in an infusion of sanicle, rue, or St. John's wort will relieve the swelling.

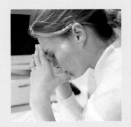

Stings

Insect bites and stings vary in seriousness, but can result in localized pain and sometimes nausea or fainting.

AROMATHERAPY For insect bites, put a drop of neat lavender oil on the place affected. For plant stings, this procedure can be repeated.

HOMEOPATHY Ledum 30c is good for insect bites where there is swelling. Apis 30c can be used for burning of the area around the bite.

HERBAL REMEDIES A fresh slice of onion applied to the sting or bite will give relief.

Bites

A bite from any animal (including another person) should receive immediate professional attention. The bite should be rinsed with plenty of cold water.

AROMATHERAPY For insect bites, put a drop of neat lavender oil on the place affected.

HOMEOPATHY Ledum 30c is good for insect bites where there is swelling. Apis 30c can be used for burning of the area around the bite.

HERBAL REMEDIES Apply fresh aloe vera sap to the insect bite. If the bite becomes infected, bathe it with echinacea or calendula tea.

Nosebleeds

Nosebleeds can result from a blow or illness, but sometimes they just occur spontaneously.

HOMEOPATHY Arnica 30c will help stop bleeding caused by a blow to the nose. Phosphorus 30c can be used for spontaneous nosebleeds in children.

HERBAL REMEDIES A traditional remedy is to insert a yarrow leaf into the nostril, and squeeze the nose gently until a blood clot forms.

Fainting

Fainting is caused by a temporary reduction in the supply of blood to the brain, and may be caused by shock, exhaustion, or an overheated atmosphere.

AROMATHERAPY Help the person to lie down and loosen their clothing, then waft some rosemary, peppermint, or basil oil under their nose.

HOMEOPATHY Ignatia 6c can be used for fainting from emotional shock. Carbo vegetabilis 6c can be used for a chilly person who collapses with cold sweats.

HERBAL REMEDIES Drinking chamomile or betony tea will aid recovery from the faint.

Glossary

A

acupressure works on same principle as acupuncture but pressure and massage are used instead of needles
acupuncture point point on the body that gives access to the meridians through which energy flows

acute describes an illness that is of sudden onset but brief duration

allergen a substance that causes an allergic reaction

allergy the body's immune system produces an abnormal response—weals, itching swelling, running eyes, difficulty with breathing—to many substances including foods, insect bites and stings, plants, house dust, and animal fur

allopathy treating a disease by inducing a condition different from the cause of the disease

anemia a deficiency in either the quality or quantity of red corpuscles in the blood

antidote term used in homeopathy to describe a remedy or substance that nullifies the effect of a prescribed remedy

asana yoga posture or position
asthma spasm of the bronchi of the lungs, narrowing the airways

aura invisible layer of energy, said to surround a human body

B

bacteria group of microorganisms, some of which cause disease

C

cartilage elastic connective tissue that forms parts of the skeleton and joint surfaces

cerebrospinal fluid clear fluid that surrounds and protects the brain and spinal cord

chakra based on the Indian understanding of energy, one of the body's energy centers

chi (qi) Chinese term for the vital energy of the universe—the life force— that permeates the body and flows along meridians

chronic describes an illness or state showing no, or extremely slow, change and persisting for a long time

coagulate the action of thickening and clotting of blood to seal wounds

complementary term used to describe alternative therapies to emphasize that they work alongside, instead of replacing, conventional medicine

compress a pad soaked in cold or hot water or infusion, applied to the body to relieve pain or swelling

contraindication a factor in a patient's condition that suggests that a particular treatment may be risky or otherwise inappropriate

D

decoction a concentrated herbal extract made by boiling woody plant material in water and then reducing the liquid

decongestant an agent for the relief or reduction of congestion, e.g. of the mucous membranes

dementia a state of serious mental deterioration

dermal sensitizer a substance that sensitizes the skin

dermal irritant a substance that irritates the skin

diagnostic tool a practice, substance, or feature that a practitioner uses to aid diagnosis

dietetics diet control and study

directive therapy therapy structured by the therapist

doshas the three organizing principles that govern mental and physical health in Ayurvedic medicine

E

electrotherapy small electric currents are passed through body to tone the system, unlock tense and painful muscles, and heal sports injuries

emetic an agent that induces vomiting, used in Ayurveda to cleanse the digestive system

endorphins group of chemicals manufactured in the brain that influence the body's response to pain

enema the injection of liquid into the rectum to cleanse the intestines

essence the integral or life-force part of a plant that is used flower remedies, herbalism, and aromatherapy

essential oil aromatic and volatile liquid obtained by expression or distillation from a single or botanical form or species of plant

F

Fight-or-flight response an automatic physiological response to a threat involving the increasing of heart rate and blood pressure in preparation for emergency action

Five elements philosophical basis of Chinese medicine that posits fire, water, wood, metal, and earth as the basic elements of the universe and hence of the human body

G

Gestalt therapy a type of psychotherapy that concentrates on a form of self-awareness, instead of treatment, where focus is on expressing immediate feelings, development of experience, and living in the moment

H

holistic medicine treatment of the whole person, mind, body, and spirit, instead of specific ailments and diseases, from the Greek word "holos," meaning whole

homeostasis in spite of varying external conditions, the internal environment of the body tends to stay constant

hormone chemical transmitter produced by the body to control the activities of specific cells

hydrotherapy use of water for special treatments, it includes showering, warm-water bathing, sea bathing, drinking, taking mineral waters at natural springs etc

hypertension raised blood pressure hypotension low blood pressure or fall of blood pressure below normal

I

immune system the body's natural means of protection from infection

immunodeficiency failure of the body's immune system to fight infection

infection multiplication of disease-producing organisms in the body

infusion extraction of herbs or other plant material by steeping in water

integrative approach using more than one type of treatment, usually of different disciplines to effect best treatment

iridology study of the colored part of the eye—the iris—to detect inner disease

J

jungian therapy form of psychotherapy based on teachings of Carl Gustav Jung (1875-1961)

K

kinesiology allergy diagnosis based on testing muscles

L

lesion change in the structure or function of bodily tissues, usually the result of disease or injury

lymph clear, colorless fluid containing white blood cells that collects in body tissue around blood vessels and is transported by the lymphatic system, playing an important role in immunity

M

maharishi a Hindu teacher of mystic and religious knowledge

mandala designs in Hindu or Buddhist art, usually circular, which symbolize the universe and are used as a focus for meditation

mantra words or sounds repeated as a focus for concentration in meditation

meridian term used in used in Chinese medicine for the pathways that carry chi, or energy, throughout the body

moxa the dried herb, *Artemesia vulgaris*, or common mugwort, burned on an acupuncture needle

moxibustion the process of heating an acupuncture needle with moxa; the warmth passes down the needle and further stimulates the acupuncture point

mother tincture used in homeopathy, the first dilution of the original substance

muskuloskeletal pertaining to the muscles and bones of the body

N

neuralgia general term for severe pain originating from a nerve

nondirective therapy therapy in which the therapist does not structure the therapy

nosode a homeopathic remedy that is made from the bacteria or virus that causes the disease

O

orthodox diagnosis Western medicine diagnosis

P

PMS premenstrual syndrome, also known as PMT or premenstrual tension

palpation examination by touch/with the hands

panchakarma Ayurvedic purifying therapy that uses various methods including enemas, purging, and nasal inhalations to cleanse the body

pediatrician medical consultant who specializes in the care of children

phobia persistent, irrational fear of some event or thing

physiotherapy treatment of injuries and disease by physical means such as massage or exercises, rather than by drugs or other medicine

phytotherapy medical treatment with herbs

pituitary gland gland in the base of the brain that produces hormones, some of which act directly on the body while others stimulate hormone production in other endocrine glands

potentization method of producing infinitesimally small dilutions of substances to use as effective medicines in homeopathy

poultice therapeutic application of a moist mass, such as a bunch of herbs, to the body to encourage local circulation and relieve pain

prana term used in yoga meaning life energy

pranayama yoga energy-expanding techniques

psyche the human mind or soul

Q

qi see chi

R

repertorize a system using charts, or a computer, to work out most suitable homeopathic remedy

repertory homeopathic reference—a comprehensive list of human ailments and their remedies

Rogerian therapy nondirective person-centered-psychotherapy developed by Carl Rogers (1902 –1987), which allows the client to feel in control

S

sanskrit classical literary language of the Hindu scriptures, dating from 1500 BCE but still in use as a sacred language today

shaman tribal priest possessing healing powers originating in Asian and in Native American societies

shock state of collapse due to a reduction in blood flow, characterized by cold sweats, dizziness, a weak pulse, and nausea, resulting from some physical or mental trauma

stimulant substance that increases activity in specific organs or systems of the body

stress the effect on a person of adverse conditions that are unavoidable, bringing about a change in the balance of hormones that may affect health and state of mind

subconscious mental processes including memories and intentions of which a person is not consciously aware but which can be accessed

sucussion process vigorous and rhythmic shaking of homeopathic dilutions that gives vigor to the remedy

symptoms perceived changes in body or mind indicating the presence of disease or injury

syndrome a combination of symptoms or signs that indicate a particular disorder

T

TCM Traditional Chinese medicine

trance altered state of awareness often associated with hypnosis

transcendental meditation movement founded by Maharishi Mahesh Yogi in 1940, based on meditation techniques instead of religious or philosophical beliefs

trauma physical injury or wound, or a psychologically disturbing experience

trigger point points of source of pain

U

ultrasound sound waves whose rapid vibrations are used in healing, especially muscles etc.

V

vibrational therapies therapies such as color therapy that treat the body on an energy level

virus minute infectious particle that can reproduce within cells

vital force another name for the life force of chi or qi

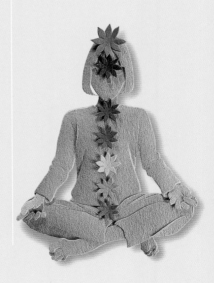

Further reading

ACUPRESSURE
Acupressure Techniques Dr. Julian Kenyon, Thorsons 1987

ACUPUNCTURE
Acupuncture for Everyone Dr. Ruth Lever, Penguin 1987
Acupuncture: A Comprehensive Text J. O'Connor & D. Bensky, Eastland Press Seattle 1981
Health Essentials: Acupuncture Peter Mole, Element Books 1992
Acupuncture Medicine Dr Y. Omara Japan: Japan Publications 1982
Traditional Acupuncture, The Law of the Five Elements Dianne Connelly, Center for Traditional Acupuncture Columbia 1979

ALEXANDER TECHNIQUE
The Alexander Technique: Natural Poise for Health, Richard Brennan, Element Books 1991
Alexander Technique C. Stevens, Optima 1987
Alexander Technique: A Practical Introduction R. Brennan, Element Books 1998
Body Learning M. Gelb, Aurum Press 1981
Health Essentials: The Alexander Technique R. Brennan, Element Books 1991

AROMATHERAPY
The Complete Illustrated Guide to Aromatherapy Julia Lawless, Element Books 1997
Aromatherapy Christine Wildwood, Element Books 1991
Aromatherapy An A-Z Patricia Davis, C.W. Daniel 1988
The Aromatherapy Book Jeanne Rose, North Atlantic Books 1994
In a Nutshell: Aromatherapy Sheila Lavery, Element Books 1997
Aromatherapy for Healing the Spirit Gabrielle Mojay, Gaia Books 1996
The Complete Aromatherapy Handbook Susanne Fischer-Rizzi, Stirling USA 1990

The Fragrant Mind Valerie Anne Worwood, Doubleday 1996
The Fragrant Pharmacy Valerie Anne Worwood, Bantam Books 1995

ART THERAPY
Art as Therapy S. McNiff, Piatkus 1994

AYURVEDA
Ayurveda Scott Gerson, Element Books 1993
Complete Illustrated Guide to Ayurveda Gopi Warrier & Dr. Deepika Gunawant, Element Books 1997
The Handbook of Ayureda D.r Shantha Godagma, Kyle Cathie 1997
Quantum Healing Dr. Deepak Chopra, Bantam Books 1989
Return of the Rishi Dr. Deepak Chopra, Houghton Mifflin Co., 1988
The Seven Pillars of Ancient Wisdom Dr. Douglas Baker, Douglas Baker Publishing, 1982
A Handbook of Ayurveda Vaida Bhagwan Dash & Acarya Manfred M. Junius, Concept Publishing Co., India 1983
Ancient Indian Massage Harish Johari, Munshiram Manoharial 1984
Basic Principles of Ayurveda Bhagwan Dash, Concept Publishing Co., India 1980

BATES METHOD
Bates Method P. Mansfield, Vermillion 1995

CHI KUNG
The Art of Chi Kung Wong Kiew Kit, Element Books 1993
Between Heaven and Earth H. Beinfield and E. Korngold, Ballantine NY 1991
Health Essentials: Chi Kung J. McRitchie, Element Books 1993

CHIROPRACTIC
Dynamic Chiropractic Today M. Copland Griffiths, Thorsons 1991

COLOR THERAPY

Color Me Healing Jack Allanach, Element Books 1997
Health Essentials: Color Therapy Pauline Wills, Element Books 1993

FELDENKRAIS METHOD

Awareness Through Movement Moshe Feldenkrais, Penguin 1990

HYDR.OTHERAPY

The Complete Book of Water Therapy Dian Dinsin Buchman, Keats 1994
Hydr.otherapy: Water and Nature C. L. Thompson, Kingston Publications 1970

HYPNOTHERAPY

Principles of Hypnotherapy Vera Peiffer, Thorsons 1996
Health Essentials: Self-Hypnosis Elaine Sheehan, Element Books 1995

MASSAGE

Massage: A Practical Introduction Stewart Mitchell, Element Books 1992
The Complete Book of Massage Clare Maxwell-Hudson, Dorling Kindersley 1988
Manipulation and Mobilisation Susan L. Edmund, Mosby 1993
The Complete Illustrated Guide to Massage Stewart Mitchell, Element Books 1997

MEDITATION

Teach Yourself Meditation James Hewitt, Hodder & Stoughton 1978
The Meditator's Handbook David Fontana, Element Books 1992
How to Meditate K. McDonald, Wisdom 1984

REFLEXOLOGY

The Complete Illustrated Guide to Reflexology Inge Dougans, Element Books 1996
The Reflexology Partnership Adamson and Harris, Kyle Cathie 1995
Reflexology: The Ancient Answer Ann Gilanders, Jenny Lee Publishing 1994
Reflexology: The Definitive Practioner's Manual Beryl Crane, Element Books 1997
Reflexology and Color Therapy: A Practical Introduction Pauline Wills, Element Books 1998

SHIATSU

The Art of Shiatsu: A Step-by-Step Guide Oliver Cowmeadow, Element Books 1992
Shiatsu: A Practical Introduction Oliver Cowmeadow, Element Books 1998
The Book of Shiatsu P. Lundberg, Gaia Books 1992
Health Essentials: Shiatsu Elaine Liechti, Element Books 1992
Shiatsu: The Complete Guide C. Jarmey & G. Mojay, Thorsons 1991
The Shiatsu Workbook N. Dawes, Piatkus Books 1991

T'AI CHI CH'UAN

The Complete Book of Tai Chi Chuan Wong Kiew Kit, Element Books 1996
The Elements of Tai Chi Paul Crompton, Element Books 1990
The Way of Energy Lam Kam Chuen, Gaia Books 1991
The Way of Harmony H. Reid, Gaia Books 1988

YOGA

The Elements of Yoga Godfrey Devereux, Element Books 1994
The Complete Yoga Course Howard Kent, Headline Press 1993
The Yoga Book Stephen Sturgess, Element Books 1997

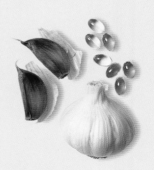

Useful addresses

ACUPUNCTURE

AMERICAN ASSOCIATION FOR
ACUPUNCTURE AND ORIENTAL
MEDICINE
4101 Lake Boone Trail
Suite 102
Raleigh
North Carolina 27607
1 919 787 5181

NATIONAL ACUPUNCTURE AND
ORIENTAL MEDICINE ALLIANCE
PO Box 77511
Seattle
Washington 98177-0531

NATIONAL COMMISSION FOR THE
CERTIFICATION OF ACUPUNCTURISTS
PO Box 97075
Washington DC 20090-7075
1 202 232 1404
fax 1 202 462 6157

ACUPUNCTURE FOUNDATION
OF CANADA
7321 Victoria Park Avenue
Unit 18
Markham
Ontario Canada
L3R 2ZB

BRITISH ACUPUNCTURE COUNCIL
63 Jeddo Road
London W12 9HQ
UK
0208 735 0400

LONDON SCHOOL OF
ACUPUNCTURE AND TRADITIONAL
CHINESE MEDICINE
60 Bunhill Row
London EC1Y 8QD
UK

BRITISH MEDICAL
ACUPUNCTURE SOCIETY
Newton House
Newton Lane
Lower Whitley
Warrington
Cheshire WA4 4JA
UK
01925 730727

NEW ZEALAND REGISTER
OF ACUPUNCTURISTS INC.
PO Box 9950
Wellington 1
New Zealand
64 4 476 8578

WESTERN CAPE SU JOK
ACUPUNCTURE INSTITUTE
3 Periwinkle Close
Kommetjie
7975 South Africa

ALEXANDER TECHNIQUE

NORTH AMERICAN SOCIETY OF
THE TEACHERS OF THE ALEXANDER
TECHNIQUE (NASTAT)
PO Box 517
Urbana
Illinois 61801-0517
1 217 367 6956

CANADIAN SOCIETY
OF THE TEACHERS OF THE
ALEXANDER TECHNIQUE
PO Box 47025
No 19-555 West 12th Avenue
Vancouver, British Columbia
Canada V5Z 3XO

SOCIETY OF TEACHERS OF
THE ALEXANDER TECHNIQUE
20 London House
266 Fulham Road
London SW10 9EL
UK
0207 351 0828

AUSTRALIAN SOCIETY OF TEACHERS
OF THE ALEXANDER TECHNIQUE
PO Box 716
Darlington
New South Wales 2010
Australia
61 8339 571

ART THERAPY

AMERICAN ART THERAPY
ASSOCIATION
1202 Allanson Road
Mundelein
Illinois 60060

NATIONAL COALITION OF
ARTS THERAPY ORGANIZATIONS
505 11th Street
South East Washington
DC 20002
1 202 543 6864

BRITISH ASSOCIATION
OF ART THERAPISTS
11a Richmond Road
Brighton BN2 3RL
UK

AYURVEDIC MEDICINE

AMERICAN ASSOCIATION
OF AYURVEDIC MEDICINE
PO Box 598
South Lancaster
Mass 01561
1 800 843 8332

MAPI INC
Garden of the Gods Business
Park
1115 Elkton Drive
Suite 401
Colorado Springs
Colorado 80907

BIOFEEDBACK: ASSOCIATION
FOR APPLIED PSYCHOPHYSIOLOGY
AND BIOFEEDBACK
10200 West 44th Avenue
Apt 304
Wheat Ridge
Colorado 80033-8436

CANADIAN ASSOCIATION
OF AYERVEIC MEDICINE
PO Box 541
Station B
Ottawa
Ontario Canada K1P 5P8
1 613 837 5737

SOUTH AFRICAN AYURVEDIC
MEDICINE ASSOCIATION
85 Harvey Road
Morningside
Durban 4001 South Africa

AYURVEDIC MEDICAL ASSOCIATION
17 Bromham Mill
Gilford Park
Milton Keynes MK14 5KP
UK
01908 617089

AYURVEDIC COMPANY OF GREAT
BRITAIN
50 Penywern Road
London SW5 9XS
UK

AYURVEDIC LIVING
PO Box 188
Exeter EX4 5AB
UK

AYURVEDIC MEDICAL ASSOCIATION
The Hale Clinic
Park Crescent
London W1N 3HE
UK

MAHARISHI AYUR-VEDA
HEALTH CENTRE
24 Linhope Street
London NW1 6HT
UK
0207 724 6267

MAHARISHI AYUR-VEDA
HEALTH CENTRE
The Golden Dome
Woodley Park
Skelmersdale WN8 6UQ
UK
01695 51008

CHI KUNG

CHI KUNG SCHOOL AT
THE BODY ENERGY CENTER
James MacRitchie & Damaris
Jarboux
PO Box 19708
Boulder
Colorado 80308
1 303 442 3131/2250

NATIONAL QIGONG (CHI KUNG)
ASSOCIATION
PO Box 20218
Boulder
Colorado 80308
1 218 984 3319

TSE QIGONG CENTRE
Qi Magazine
PO Box 116
Manchester M20 3YN
UK

QIGONG ACADEMY
8103 Marlborough Avenue
Cleveland
Ohio 44129

WORLD ACADEMIC SOCIETY
OF MEDICAL QIGONG
No 11 Heping Jie Nei Kou
Beijing 100029 China

QIGONG ASSOCIATION
OF AUSTRALIA
458 White Horse Road
Surrey Hills
Victoria 3127 Australia
61 3 9836 6961
fax 61 3 830 5608

DR. YVES REQUENA
Institut Euopeen de Qi Gong
La Ferme des Vences
13122 Ventabren France

CHIROPRACTIC

AMERICAN CHIROPRACTIC
ASSOCIATION
1701 Clarendon Boulevard
Arlington
Virginia 22201
1 703 276 8800

INTERNATIONAL CHIROPRACTORS'
ASSOCIATION
Suite 1000
1110 North Glebe Road
Arlington
Virginia 22201
1 703 528 5000

WORLD CHIROPRACTIC ALLIANCE
2950 North Dobson Road
Suite One
Chandler
Arizona 85224-1802
1 800 347 1011

CANADIAN CHIROPRACTIC
ASSOCIATION
1396 Eglinton Avenue West
Toronto
Ontario Canada M6C 2E4
1 416 781 5656

BRITISH ASSOCIATION FOR
APPLIED CHIROPRACTIC
The Old Post Office
Cherry Street
Stratton Audley
Bicester OX6 9BA
UK

BRITISH CHIROPRACTIC
ASSOCIATION
Blagrave House
Blagrave Street
Reading RG1 1QB
UK
0118 950 5950

CHIROPRACTIC ASSOCIATION
OF IRELAND
28 Fair Street
Drogheda
County Louth
Irish Republic
353 41 305999

CHIROPRACTIC ASSOCIATION
Box 23
Tanglin Post Office
Singapore
65 293 9843/ 734 8584

CHIROPRACTIC COUNCIL OF JAPAN
2621-5
Noborito Tama-ku
Kawasaki 214
Japan
fax 81 44 933 4449

HONG KONG CHIROPRACTORS'
ASSOCIATION
GPO Box 5588
Hong Kong
852 375 5785
fax 852 537 5487

MANU R SHAH D C
Sheikh Ismail Building
Aquem Alto
Margao
Goa 403 601 India
91 83 422 3707

CHIROPRACTORS' ASSOCIATION
OF AUSTRALIA
PO Box 241
Springwood
New South Wales 2777
Australia
61 47 515 644
fax 61 47 515 856

NEW ZEALAND
CHIROPRACTORS' ASSOCIATION
PO Box 7144
Wellesley Street
Auckland New Zealand
64 9 373 4343
fax 64 373 5973

COGNITIVE THERAPY

ASSOCIATION OF COGNITIVE
ANALYTIC THERAPISTS
4th Floor North Wing
Division of Academic Psychiatry
St.Thomas's Hospital
London SE1 7EH
UK
0207 928 9292 x 3769

BRITISH ASSOCIATION FOR
BEHAVIOURAL AND COGNITIVE
PSYCHOTHERAPIES
Dept of Clinical Psychology
Northwick Park Hospital
Watford Road
Harrow HA1 3UJ
UK
0208 869 2325

COLOR THERAPY

COLOUR AND REFLEXOLOGY
9 Wyndale Avenue
Kingsbury
London NW9 9PT
UK
0208 204 7672

DANCE THERAPY

AMERICAN DANCE
THERAPY ASSOCIATION
2000 Century Plaza
Suite 108
Columbia
Maryland 21044
1 410 997 4040

INTERNATIONAL DANCE EXERCISE
ASSOCIATION (IDEA)
6190 Cornerstone Court East
Apt 204
San Diego
California 92121-3773
1 619 535 8979

LABAN CENTRE FOR
MOVEMENT AND DANCE
Laurie Grove
New Cross
London SE14 6NH
UK
0208 692 4070

HYPNOTHERAPY

AMERICAN ASSOCIATION OF
PROFESSIONAL HYPNOTHERAPISTS
PO Box 29
Boones Mill
Virginia 24065
1 703 334 3035

NATIONAL SOCIETY
OF HYPNOTHERAPISTS
2175 North West 86th
Suite 6A
Des Moines
Iowa 50325
1 515 270 2280

BRITISH SOCIETY OF EXPERIMENTAL
AND CLINICAL HYPNOSIS
c/o Dept. of Psychology
Grimsby General Hospital
Scartle Road
Grimsby DN33 2BA
UK
01472 874 111

BRITISH SOCIETY OF MEDICAL
AND DENTAL HYPNOSIS
17 Keppelview Road
Kimberworth
Rotherham S61 2 AR
UK
01709 554558

BRITISH HYPNOTHERAPY
ASSOCIATION
67 Upper Berkeley Street
London W1H 7DH
UK
0207 723 4443

MASSAGE THERAPY

AMERICAN MASSAGE
THERAPY ASSOCIATION
820 Davis Street
Suite 100
Evanston
Illinois 60201-4444
1 847 864 0123

NATIONAL ASSOCIATION
OF MASSAGE THERAPY
PO Box 1400
Westminster
Colorado 80030-1400
1 800 776 6268

BRITISH MASSAGE
THERAPY COUNCIL
Greenbank House
65a Adelphi Street
Preston PR1 7BH
UK
01772 881063

MASSAGE THERAPY INSTITUTE
OF GREAT BRITAIN
PO Box 27/26
London NW2 4NR
UK
0208 208 1607

LONDON COLLEGE OF MASSAGE
5 Newman Passage
London W1P 3PF
UK
0207 323 3574

SOCIETY OF CLINICAL MASSEURS
PO Box 483
9 Delhi Street
Mitchum 3131
Victoria Australia
61 3 874 6973

MEDITATION

SCHOOL OF MEDITATION
158 Holland Park Avenue
London W11 4UH
UK
0207 603 6116

TRANSCENDENTAL MEDITATION
Freepost
London SW1P 4YY
UK

MUSIC THERAPY

AMERICAN ASSOCIATION
OF MUSIC THERAPY
PO Box 80012
Valley Forge
Pennsylvania 19484

NATIONAL ASSOCIATION
OF MUSIC THERAPY
8455 Colesville Road
Suite 1000
Silver Springs
Maryland 20910
1 301 589 3300

BRITISH SOCIETY FOR
MUSIC THERAPY
25 Rosslyn Avenue
East Barnet EN4 8DH
UK
0208 368 8879

OSTEOPATHY

AMERICAN ACADEMY
OF OSTEOPATHY
3500 DePauw Boulevard
Suite 1080
Indianapolis
Indiana 46268-1136
1 317 879 1881

AMERICAN ASSOCIATION
OF COLLEGES OF
OSTEOPATHIC MEDICINE
6110 Executive Boulevard
Apt 405
Rockville
Maryland 20852
1 301 468 0990

AMERICAN OSTEOPATHIC
ASSOCIATION
142 East Ontario Street
Chicago
Illinois 60611
1 312 280 5800
fax 1 312 202 8200

OSTEOPATHIC
INFORMATION SERVICE
PO Box 2074
Reading
Berkshire RG1 4YR
UK

GENERAL REGISTER AND
COUNCIL OF OSTEOPATHS
56 London Street
Reading
Berkshire RG1 4SQ
UK

NSW CHIROPRACTORS AND
OSTEOPATHIC REGISTRATION
BOARD
PO Box K599
Haymarket
New South Wales 2000
Australia
61 2 281 0884
fax 61 2 281 2030

PSYCHOTHERAPY

UK COUNCIL FOR PSYCHOTHERAPY
167-9 Great Portland Street
London WIN 5FB
UK
0207 436 3002

EUROPEAN ASSOCIATION
FOR PSYCHOTHERAPY
Rosenbursenstrasse
8/3/7
A-1010 Vienna
Austria
43 1 512 7090

REFLEXOLOGY

REFLEXOLOGY ASSOCIATION OF
AMERICA
4012 S. Rainbow Boulevard
Box K585
Las Vegas
Nevada 89103-2509

REFLEXOLOGY ASSOCIATION OF
CANADA (RAC)
11 Glen Cameron Road
Unit 4
Thornhill
Ontario L8T 4NB Canada
1 905 889 5900

BRITISH REFLEXOLOGY ASSOCIATION
Monks Orchard
Whitbourne
Worcester WR6 5RB
UK
01886 821 207

ASSOCIATION OF REFLEXOLOGISTS
27 Old Gloucester Street
London WC1N 3XX
UK

BRITISH SCHOOL OF
REFLEXOLOGY AND HOLISTIC
ASSOCIATION OF REFLEXOLOGISTS
92 Sheering Road
Old Harlow
Essex CM17 0JW
UK
01279 429060

INTERNATIONAL FEDERATION
OF REFLEXOLOGISTS
76-8 Edridge Road
Croydon
Surrey CR0 1EF
UK
0208 667 9458
fax 0208 649 9291

IRISH REFLEXOLOGISTS INSTITUTE
c/o 11 Fitzwilliam Place
Dublin 2

Irish Republic
353 1 760137

CHINA REFLEXOLOGY ASSOCIATION
PO Box 2002
Beijing 100026 China

NEW ZEALAND REFLEXOLOGY
ASSOCIATION
PO Box 31 084
Auckland 4
New Zealand

REFLEXOLOGY ASSOCIATION OF
AUSTRALIA
15 Kedumba Crescent
Turramurra 2074
New South Wales Australia

SHIATSU

AMERICAN SHIATSU ASSOCIATION
PO Box 718
Jamaica Plain
Massachusetts 02130

THE SHIATSU SOCIETY OF
GREAT BRITAIN
5 Foxcote
Workingham
Berkshire RG11 3PG
UK

SHIATSU SOCIETY
31 Pullman Lane
Godalming
Surrey GU7 1XY
UK

SHIATSU THERAPY ASSOCIATION OF
AUSTRALIA
PO Box 1
Balaclava
Victoria 3183 Australia
61 03 530 0067

T'AI CHI

T'AI CHI UNION FOR
GREAT BRITAIN
102 Felsham Road
London SW15 1 DQ
UK

WORLD T'AI CHI BOXING
ASSOCIATION
1 Deans Way
London N2 0NF UK
0208 264 8074
www.taiji.net
paul@taiji.net

YOGA

INTERNATIONAL YOGA TEACHERS'
ASSOCIATION
c/o 14-15 Huddart Avenue
Normanhurst
New South Wales 2076
Australia
61 2 9484 9848

UNITY IN YOGA
303 2495 West 2nd Avenue
Vancouver
British Columbia Canada
VGK 1J5

BRITISH WHEEL OF YOGA
1 Hamilton Place
Boston Road
Sleaford
Lincolnshire NG34 7ES
UK
01529 306851
fax 01529 303233

THE IYENGAR YOGA INSTITUTE
223a Randolf Avenue
Maida Vale
London W9 1NL
UK
0207 624 3080

SIVANANDA YOGA VEDANTA
CENTRE
51 Felsham Road
London SW15 1AZ
UK

BKS IYENGAR ASSOCIATION OF
AUSTRALIA
1 Rickman Avenue
Mosman 2088
New South Wales Australia

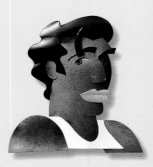

List of contributors

ACUPUNCTURE
Mike Cummings
is Director of Education for the British Medical Acupuncture Society. He served as a GP in the Royal Air Force for nearly seven years before taking over a private acupuncture practice in the southwest of England. He has worked as Director of Education for the British Medical Acupuncture Society for many years.

ALEXANDER TECHNIQUE
Sabrina Kiefer
A dancer in her teens and later a journalist, Sabrina Kiefer first used the Alexander Technique herself to overcome a chronic back problem. She has been an Alexander teacher since 1996, and sits on the governing council of the Society of Teachers of the Alexander Technique. Her practice is in London.

AROMATHERAPY
Helen Farmer-Knowles
is an aromatherapist, counselor, electrocrystal therapy practitioner, advisor on essential oils to the Institute of Complementary Medicine, and author of *The Garden Healer*. For some years she has been an independent researcher into health benefits of herbal plants and their essential oils, for both humans and animals.

ART THERAPY
Francesca Raphael
originally trained as a counselor before becoming an art therapist. She has worked both in the National Health Service with the adult mentally ill and in the voluntary sector with adolescents and young adults. She spent many years developing and teaching an integrative arts psychotherapy training course before going on to further training herself as a psychoanalytic psychotherapist. She works both as an art psychotherapist and psychoanalytic therapist in private practice.

AYURVEDA
Donn Brennan
qualified in medicine in 1979, and then worked in hospital medicine and general practice for ten years. In 1981 he qualified as a teacher of TM, and from 1984–85 did 18 months training in the US and India on Maharishi Ayurveda. Since 1990 he has traveled throughout Britain, Ireland, and Iceland consulting and lecturing to the public and the medical profession on transcendental meditation and Maharishi Ayurveda.

CHI KUNG
Paul Brecher
has over 20 years of experience in the martial arts and is senior instructor for the World Tai Chi Boxing Association in London. He has written numerous articles and given Tai Chi demonstrations on television. He is author of *The Principles of Tai Chi* and *The Way of The Spiritual Warrior*. He is also a qualified practitioner of acupuncture and traditional Chinese herbal medicine, treating patients at his private clinic in London.

CHIROPRACTIC
Mike Barber
graduated from the Anglo-European College of Chiropractic in Bournemouth in 1977. After having worked as a clinic associate for four years in Leeds, he returned to his home town of Sheffield, setting up the highly successful Sheffield Chiropractic Clinic. After starting a Masters degree in Clinical Chiropractic, Mike initiated a Spinal Rehabilitation Centre within the clinic. Mike now runs his own clinic in South Wales, and has recently been elected president of the British Chiropractic Association.

COLOR THERAPY
Jan Davidson
has worked with color therapy for well over 20 years, first as a chromo practitioner and then, due to demand for high quality training, as a trainer. She has run the internationally known College of Chromo Therapy (CTT) for the last ten years. Jan is also a consultant to industry and commerce on color psychology.

DANCE THERAPY
Laurence Higgens
trained in dance movement therapy at Laban Centre, London and worked in the National Health Service at Springfield Hospital, London for eight years. He is Course Leader of the MA professional training program at Laban Centre and also works in private practice. A past chair of the Association for Dance Movement Therapy, UK, he currently serves on the Council, and on the Education and Training Committees of the Association.

HEALING
Michael Dibdin
retired from merchant banking in 1986 to develop a new career in hypnotherapy and counseling. A chance encounter prompted him take a serious interest in healing. He has organized the Doctor-Healer

Network, an informal group of doctors, nurses and other health professionals, scientific researchers, and healers who have worked with the medical profession, since 1995. Now with some 150 members, its aim is to make healing better understood among the medical profession. He is also involved in the management of the Confederation of Healing Organizations.

HERBAL MEDICINE
Peter Conway-Grim
is a practicing medical herbalist and a member of both the National Institute of Medical Herbalists and the College of Practitioners of Phytotherapy. He is director of the London Clinic of Phytotherapy, the main training clinic for students studying with the College of Phytotherapy. With his partner Catherine Craig, he runs a private herbal practice in Edinburgh. He is a former coeditor of the *European Journal of Herbal Medicine* and current editor of the *British Journal of Phytotherapy*.

HOMEOPATHY
Anne E.Feist
has been a practicing homeopath since 1987, having studied, qualified, and registered with the General Council and Register of Consultant Herbalists and

Homeopaths (now known as IRCH). She also became a qualified iridologist in 1991 and was made a fellow of the Guild of Naturopathic Iridologists in 1996. She qualified as a vega allergy analyst in 1997 and has a busy practice, using all three disciplines, in Ninfield, East Sussex.

HYPNOTHERAPY
John Butler
has been a practicing hypnotherapist and psychotherapist for over 20 years. His approach is integrative and he works with both long- and short-term clients. He is a university lecturer in psychology and is also an experienced trainer and supervisor of hypnotherapists and psychotherapists. He has contributed to many publications and has taken part in radio and television broadcasts. He is a registered psychotherapist with the United Kingdom Council of Psychotherapy and has served on its Governing Board.

MASSAGE
Caroline Stevenson
is a Holistic Health Consultant and Practitioner. She has a degree in social work and is a registered nurse. She is also qualified to practice in a range of complementary therapies including iridology,

acupuncture, aromatherapy, massage, shiatsu and reiki. Caroline has been involved in complementary medicine for over 20 years.

MEDITATION
Kai Kermani

is a member of most of the major Royal Medical Colleges and was a holistic general practitioner until accidentally blinded nine years ago. He now devotes his life to using his gifts to empower and inspire people to transform their lives and heal themselves. Dr. Kermani is also a counselor, stress management consultant, Autogenic Trainer and therapist, lectures widely, and facilitates his Inspirational Healing Workshops internationally. He has appeared on television and radio, written numerous articles on health issues, also contributed to many books, and is the author of the highly successful book *Autogenic Training*.

MUSIC
Helen Tyler

is a music therapist and Assistant Director of the Nordoff-Robbins Music Therapy Centre in North London. She had wide experience of teaching music in schools at all levels from nursery age upward before training

as a music therapist. She lectures extensively and has published several articles about music therapy.

NATUROPATHY
Ian P. Drysdale

is a registered osteopath and registered naturopath with a B.Sc (Hons) in biochemistry/physiology from Queen Elizabeth College, London (1971). He studied for his Ph.D in clinical endocrinology (biochemistry) at the Royal Postgraduate Medical School and Northwick Park Hospital and has since taken the ND, DO course program at the British College of Naturopathy and Osteopathy. He first began lecturing at the BCNO in 1971 and has remained associated with the College ever since. He has been its Principal since 1990.

OSTEOPATHY
Ian P. Drysdale

is a registered osteopath and registered naturopath with a BSc (Hons) in biochemistry/physiology from Queen Elizabeth College, London (1971). He studied for his PhD in clinical endocrinology (biochemistry) at the Royal Postgraduate Medical School and Northwick Park Hospital and has since taken the ND, DO course programme at the British College of Naturopathy

and Osteopathy. He first began lecturing at the BCNO in 1971 and has remained associated with the College ever since. He has been its Principal since 1990.

PSYCHOTHERAPY
John Butler

has been a practising hypnotherapist and psychotherapist for over 20 years. His approach is integrative and he works with both long- and short-term clients. He is a university lecturer in psychology and is also an experienced trainer and supervisor of hypnotherapists and psychotherapists. He has contributed to many publications and has taken part in radio and television broadcasts. He is a registered psychotherapist with the United Kingdom Council of Psychotherapy and has served on its Governing Board.

REFLEXOLOGY
Hazel Goodwin

taught in secondary schools in England and Africa for 20 years before training as a yoga teacher in the 1970s. She then worked for some years with emotionally disturbed teenagers and psychiatric patients. She took courses in massage, sports injury, and aromatherapy before discovering reflexology. She joined the

Association of Reflexologists (AoR) in 1985, shortly after qualifying, and in 1990 helped to set up a working party to develop training standards for reflexology practitioners. Hazel was chairperson of the AoR from 1993 to 1999 and is currently the Association's president. She has written a Reflexology Workbook and many articles on complementary medicine.

RELAXATION
Kai Kermani
is a member of most of the major Royal Medical Colleges and was a holistic GP until accidentally blinded. He now devotes his life to using his gifts to empower and inspire people to transform their lives and heal themselves. Dr Kermani is also a counsellor, stress management consultant, Autogenic Trainer and therapist, lectures widely and facilitates his Inspirational Healing Workshops internationally. He has appeared on television and radio, written numerous articles on health issues, also contributed to many books, and is the author of the highly successful book *Autogenic Training*.

SHIATSU
Katharine Hall
traveled to China in 1986,

where her interest in Oriental philosophy, art, and medicine developed. In 1988 she returned to the UK to study at The Shiatsu College and became a registered practitioner in 1991. She has an established Shiatsu practice in London, teaches and works in political and international liaison for the Shiatsu Society UK.

TAI CHI
Paul Brecher
has over 20 years of experience in the martial arts and is senior instructor for the World Tai Chi Boxing Association in London. He has written numerous articles and given Tai Chi demonstrations on television. He is author of *The Principles of Tai Chi* and *The Way of The Spiritual Warrior*. He is also a qualified practitioner of acupuncture and traditional chinese herbal medicine, treating patients at his private clinic in Hampstead, London, and can be contacted on 0181 264 8074.

TRADITIONAL CHINESE MEDICINE
Sue Seddon
is a writer and editor with many years experience of complementary therapies. She is a qualified teacher and has studied Art Therapy in Edinburgh.

VISUALIZATION
Kai Kermani
is a member of most of the major Royal Medical Colleges and was a holistic GP until accidentally blinded. He now devotes his life to using his gifts to empower and inspire people to transform their lives and heal themselves. Dr Kermani is also a counsellor, stress management consultant, Autogenic Trainer and therapist, lectures widely and facilitates his Inspirational Healing Workshops internationally. He has appeared on television and radio, written numerous articles on health issues, also contributed to many books, and is the author of *Autogenic Training*.

YOGA
Sue Seddon
is a writer and editor with many years experience of complementary therapies. She is a qualified teacher and has studied Art Therapy in Edinburgh.

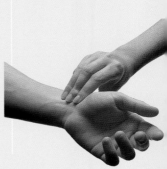

Index

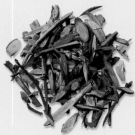

Acknowledgments

The publishers are grateful to the following for permission to reproduce copyright material.

AKG, London: p134

A-Z Botanical Collection: pp57B, 61L, 87, 165T

Bridgeman Art Library: pp29 (Chester Beatty Library, Dublin), 34 (Lambeth Palace Library, London), 79 (Ashmolean Museum, Oxford), 83 (Giraudon, Paris), 98T (National Museum, Seoul), 128 (Galleria dell'Accademia, Florence), 140 (Bibliotheque Nationale, Paris), 146 (British Library, London)

Bruce Coleman: pp135C, 142

British Chiropractic Association: p168

British School of Osteopathy: p174

e.t. archive: p12

Hulton Getty Picture Collection: p30

Hutchison Library: p31B

Image Bank: pp2, opp. 11, 17CL, 19C, 21C, 22L, 32, 56C, 57C, 94, opp. 97, 99, opp. 109, 115, 116C, 135L&B, 141, 164, 165B, 169, 171C, 173, 176T, 177, opp. 179, 189

Images Colour Library: p119

Rex Features: p98B

Science Photo Library: pp24, 36T, 52, 54, 116B, 132, opp. 145, opp. 167, 170, 171R, 175, 182

Stock Market: opp. p35

Society of Teachers of the Alexander Technique: p36B

Tony Stone Images: pp114, 120, 122

Trip/Viesti Collection: p21B

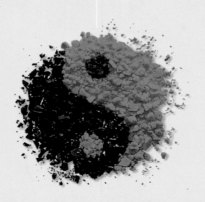